Doris Schlömmer

'Between the fronts'

Doris Schlömmer

'Between the fronts'

End-of-life care in long-term inpatient care from the perspective of nursing students

ScienciaScripts

Imprint
Any brand names and product names mentioned in this book are subject to trademark, brand or patent protection and are trademarks or registered trademarks of their respective holders. The use of brand names, product names, common names, trade names, product descriptions etc. even without a particular marking in this work is in no way to be construed to mean that such names may be regarded as unrestricted in respect of trademark and brand protection legislation and could thus be used by anyone.

Cover image: www.ingimage.com

This book is a translation from the original published under ISBN 978-620-2-21454-4.

Publisher:
Sciencia Scripts
is a trademark of
Dodo Books Indian Ocean Ltd. and OmniScriptum S.R.L publishing group

120 High Road, East Finchley, London, N2 9ED, United Kingdom
Str. Armeneasca 28/1, office 1, Chisinau MD-2012, Republic of Moldova, Europe
Managing Directors: Ieva Konstantinova, Victoria Ursu
info@omniscriptum.com

Printed at: see last page
ISBN: 978-620-8-83531-6

Abstract

Background: The care of the dying increasingly takes place in extramural long-term care facilities and leads to the institutionalisation of dying and death. Nowadays, students in health care and nursing have hardly any experience and are usually only confronted with the phenomenon of death during their training.

Aim: The question of how students experience their role as carers of dying people in inpatient long-term care facilities was investigated. The aim was to identify those aspects that can have a positive or negative influence on the experience. The qualitatively collected data was selected, categorised and interpreted using May- ring's structured content analysis.

Results: Dealing with dying and death represents an emotional burden and nursing challenge for the trainees, especially if there is insufficient support. The dissonance and subjective overload is expressed in grief, fear and helplessness and is favoured by the relationship work and an unsatisfactory working culture. The opportunity for personal dialogue and needs-oriented care in the context of support are perceived as relieving.

Outlook: End-of-life care is characterised by dignity and respect. This approach must be taught and exemplified during training. The experiences gained during training lead to the formation of empathic attitudes and the development of emotional competence. Carers must integrate trainees into the care process, argue their decisions and communicate emotions in their experiences.

Keywords: dying, end-of-life care, geriatric care facilities, nursing training.

Contents

CHAPTER 1

Introduction

Dying and death are omnipresent and present in society, but are nevertheless repeatedly tabooed, as the end of life is at odds with reality. In nursing training, an encounter with dying and death can occur suddenly and unprepared. Although trainees take on the role of carers, they are often laypeople when it comes to dealing with dying people.

1.1 Initial situation

Dying today is increasingly taking place in institutions (Nagele & Feichtner 2012; Seeger, 2011). In Europe, 20% of people die in retirement and nursing homes. The short length of stay, the high age of admission and the lack of social networks are cited as reasons for institutionalisation (DGP, 2012; Rest, 2006). This is due on the one hand to increasing life expectancy and on the other hand to the lack of care being provided at home (Statistik Austria, 2014; Giese, 2013; Wilkening & Kunz, 2003). In addition to hospitals, inpatient long-term care facilities in particular are experiencing a sharp increase as places where people die (Dasch et al., 2015; Engelke, 2015).

For trainees, the first contact in the care of terminally ill, multimorbid, very elderly residents can lead to emotional stress, psychological stress symptoms and personal consternation (Gerhard, 2015; Seeger, 2011; Jenull et al., 2008; Heller, 2007). This results in uncertainties in the encounter and challenges in care (Engelke, 2015; Ohlrogge, 2012; Widegger, 2011; Halfpap, 2009; Aulbert, 2007).

Moreover, little attention is paid to their own knowledge of the phenomenon of death and their personal experiences (Widegger et al., 2011; Student et al., 2004). Trainees have their own ideas or ideas acquired through the media and therefore have a different view of dying and death in the professional setting (Fischer, 2001, cited in Grigoleit, 2011, p. 30). Furthermore, socialisation-related, personal attitudes often remain unquestioned and are hardly reflected upon (Schwarz-Govaers, 2005, p. 38).

Caring and communicative processes are characterised by emotions, whether intentional or unintentional, and have a lasting effect on personality development in the context of lived experiences (Ohlrogge, 2012; Handler, 2013; Andraschko, 2008;). One's own affectedness manifests itself in helplessness, uncertainty, fear, anger and shock (Mutto et al., 2010; Kiger, 1994; Schleich, 1998; cited in Ohlrogge, 2012; Müller et al., 2010; Cooper & Barnett, 2005; Stähli, 2004). The burden of emotional labour and emotional dissonance are observed by Widegger et al. (2011), particularly in very young carers.

In order to be able to provide professional end-of-life care, it is necessary to deal with one's own ideas and convey an appropriate attitude and work culture during training (Jafari et al., 2015; Ek et al., 2014). However, international research findings show that nursing students are often not at all or only inadequately prepared for working with terminally ill and dying patients during their training (Araujo et al. 2004; Brisley & Wood 2004).

1.2 Objective

The aim of this study is to analyse end-of-life care in long-term inpatient care from the perspective of general health and nursing trainees. To this end, the experiences during the care and support of dying people in retirement and nursing homes are empirically analysed and subsequently challenging and stressful circumstances are presented.

The thesis aims to contribute to reducing the research gap in the field of palliative care in the context of nursing education by taking a closer look at the experience of end-of-life care. The aim of this study is not to evaluate end-of-life care in the institutions, but to identify those factors, which are perceived by the trainees as relevant in their dealings.

The following research questions are generated on the basis of the stated problem and objectives:

> How do nursing students in their role as carers experience caring for the dying in the extramural setting of retirement and nursing homes?

Which personal aspects and environmental factors can be stressful or relieving for the experience of dying and death in the inpatient long-term care sector?

1.3 Methodology

The present study is based on a defined problem description of the experience of end-of-life care in the extramural setting among nursing students in the senior healthcare and nursing service. In order to answer the central questions, the methodology of literature work, consisting of literature research and literature analysis, is chosen in the first step. In order to show the current state of research, a systematic literature search is carried out using keyword searches with the keywords dying, end-of-life care, care facilities for the elderly, nursing training in the scientific databases PUBMED and CINAHL from December 2016 to April 2017.

In German-speaking countries, only a few specific results are available; internationally, there are valid results, although these were mostly collected in the acute inpatient and long-term inpatient care sectors. It should be borne in mind that the experience and personal approach to dying are characterised by the respective culture and are therefore not comparable.

To emphasise the topicality of the available results, the search is limited to the period of the last 15 years and the Boolean operators "AND" and "NOT" are used in the online search (Behrens & Langer, 2004, p. 95).

In addition, the references of the literature used and relevant literature sources researched by hand search are also included. In the second step, the literature is systematically analysed with regard to the presentation of theory-related aspects and answers to the research question and evaluated according to criteria (Behrens & Langer, 2004, p. 131 ff.). A qualitative research approach is chosen for the empirical data collection, the aim of which is to describe the subjective views and emotional experiences of trainees in end-of-life care.

CHAPTER 2

Theoretical frame of reference

In the first part of the thesis, the terms dying and death are explained and end-of-life care is explicated in the context of the nursing profession, the institution of retirement and nursing homes and training in healthcare and nursing. It concludes by highlighting structural and personal stress factors in the confrontation with dying residents of long-term care facilities.

2.1 Dying and death

Dying is a part of human life and should be seen as a natural process at the end of life. Death represents the inevitable end. In the following, both terms are differentiated and contrasted in their perspectives.

Dying defines a period of life that precedes the time of death as the end, but whose beginning cannot be concretised (Rest, 2006, p. 18). The processual course of this period consists of different phases that the dying person goes through and perceives individually in terms of time and perception. The German palliative care physician Ingeborg Jonen-Thielemann divides the process of dying into "preterminal phase, terminal phase and state in extremis" (Jonen-Thielemann, 1997, cited in Feichtner, 2014, p. 51). The phases are defined by the state of consciousness of the dying person (cf. Jonen-Thielemann, 1997, cited in Bethmann, 2008, p. 6). Nagele & Feichtner (2005) describe that the so-called "terminal phase" begins when a person is recognised as dying. However, there are no explicit characteristics as to when the dying phase actually begins (Nagele & Feichtner, 2005, p. 37 f.).

In contrast to dying, death represents an actual, tangible point in time at the end of life, which, however, is presented differently depending on social and cultural norms (May, 2011, p. 23). On a societal-social level, death is seen in the context of immortality; on a biological-medical level, it is understood as the cessation of essential organ functions. On the philosophical-theological level, death definitively ends active, physical and spiritual existence and is thus seen as a transition to another state (Engelke, 2015, p. 22). In terms of the types of death, a distinction is made between social, psychological, clinical and biological death. The latter means the end of all organ and cell functions and thus represents the complete disintegration of all body cells of the entire organism (May, 2011, p. 23).

People in the middle of life rarely confront the idea of dying and death. As a result, they even avoid institutions such as retirement or nursing homes (Borasio, 2012; Wilkening & Kunz, 2003). It is also claimed that death was dealt with better in the last century. Engelke (2015, p. 30 ff.), however, emphasises that even before the 19th century, death was often perceived as an enemy or threat and dying people were isolated from society. Engelke (2015, p. 44) also states that caring for dying people was never a matter of course. The attitude shown to seriously ill, elderly and dying people has always been decisive in dealing with dying and death.

Demographic developments should also be taken into account in the discussion on socialisation in dealing with the dying (DGP, 2010). Due to changes in family situations, such as the employment of all family members or the generations' own living conditions, dying at home is often no longer possible or only possible under difficult conditions (Gro- nemeyer, 2002, cited in Pleschberger, 2005, p. 10). Due to this lack of confrontation, young people undoubtedly also deal less and less with dying and death and react with excessive demands and powerlessness when being accompanied (Pleschberger, 2005, p. 10; Student et al., 2004).

2.2 End-of-life care

End-of-life care is also defined as assisted dying and refers to "help with dying or for the dying person" (Rest, 2006, p. 18). The National Ethics Council (2006, p. 53) links assisted dying with "[...] measures for the care and support of the terminally ill and dying." The encounter with dying and death is seen as a task for the nursing profession and, in a broader sense, also as a professional self-image. However, this raises the question of whether and how this can be experienced and lived at all.

2.2.1 End-of-life care as a professional self-image

The professional self-image as an identity feature of carers is defined on the one hand by the carers themselves and on the other hand by the job profile required by society. In the context of end-of-life care, in addition to the carer's own identity, the social expectation that carers should be able to cope with emotional demands is taken for granted (Stöhr & Trumpetter, 2006, p. 1 f.).

For Pleschberger and Heimerl (2005), "the accompaniment, care and support of seriously ill and dying people is one of the core tasks of nursing". End-of-life care is also not bound to an institution; on the contrary, it should visualise an appropriate attitude and make all those involved responsible (Pleschberger & Heimerl, 2005, p. 15).

Caregivers should focus on the needs of those affected, express their feelings and allow closeness, even if structural and organisational conditions do not permit the necessary individualisation (Lexa, 2011, p. 20). In addition, it is important to show empathy and compassion, to overcome crises and to consider the question of meaning and spirituality. The most important points here are understanding the role model and reflecting on the feelings of the counsellor. Professional closeness creates satisfaction through relationships and should be seen as part of the caring profession (Lexa, 2011, p. 22). Carers should allow themselves to be touched by the suffering of others and surrender to their own feelings. Professional closeness also plays an important role for Öhlen et al. (2002, cited in Feichtner, 2016, p. 24) and Beatty (2013). They postulate compassion, human affection, presence and continuity.

Carers demand this closeness as a matter of course and sometimes cite it as a reason for choosing their profession: "I can and should be close to people - after all, that's why I originally started my helping profession" (Kränzle, 2011, p. 48). Similarly, accompanying the dying requires "[...] a professional approach while maintaining humanity and empathy [...]" (Widegger et al. (2011, quoted from Handler, 2014, p. 212). This requirement necessitates appropriate behaviour, but cannot always be taken for granted in terms of professional identity (Bischoff-Wanner, 2002).

Since nursing students often only come into contact with dying and death during their training, this is where they experience their first emotional challenges. Lampert (2011) considers an empathetic approach to be absolutely essential and denies that distance must be learnt during training in order to counteract emotional stress. In addition to Lampert (2011), Bischoff-Wanner (2002) also emphasises that empathy and sensitivity must be developed and promoted during training (Bischoff-Wanner, 2002, cited in Widegger et al., 2011, p. 103).

Furthermore, carers must not be allowed to get to the point where they no longer face their feelings or do not dare to admit their powerlessness. On the contrary, behaviour towards the dying requires openness and confrontation with the psychological and social situation of the person concerned (En- gelke, 2015, p. 218 ff.).

2.2.2 End-of-life care in a nursing context

Professional end-of-life care requires knowledge of basic human needs based on A. Maslow's theory of needs (Maslow, 1943, cited in Boeree, 2006, p. 4). The physiological needs, such as maintaining breathing, the desire for sleep, quenching thirst and freedom from pain, form the basis of nursing actions. With regard to the need for security, the availability of trusted persons, good care, the maintenance of personal habits and protection from physical suffering should be mentioned. In the need for love, the person concerned wants to share their worries and feelings, maintain social contacts and feel touched. He/she wants to feel like a human being and be honoured, considered and respected as a person (Rest, 2006, p. 182).

The tasks involved in end-of-life care are therefore not limited to nursing measures, but rather involve the holistic recognition of all needs, which in turn requires appropriate sensitivity and competence on the part of the people involved (DGP, 2012).

The European Association for Palliative Care (EAPC) considers the fulfilment of physical, psychological, social and spiritual needs to be core competencies of professional end-of-life care. In addition to professional competence as a professional requirement profile, social competence in particular plays a role in the core competences of palliative care (Krumm et al., 2015, p. 159). The National Ethics Council also emphasises the importance of observing and considering the above-mentioned dimensions in its statements (BGM, 2000; National Ethics Council, 2006, p. 48). As a result, intensive communication and interactive relationship work are at the centre of all nursing activities (Krumm et al., 2015, p. 162).

Nursing interventions include personal hygiene, the alleviation of thirst and pain, anxiety and respiratory distress, but also psychosocial care through congruent support and open dialogue. All measures must be carried out with a focus on self-determination and dignity (National Ethics Council, 2006, p. 53).

The fundamental objectives of end-of-life care include respect for the dignity of the dying person, as well as respecting and recognising the person as an individual. The Charter for the Care of the Critically Ill and Dying in Germany demands that "[...] every person has a right to die in dignified conditions. The dying person must be able to trust that their wishes and values will be respected (DGP, 2012). David Kessler counts dignity as one of the 12 rights of the dying and emphasises that [...] "Everyone has the right to die peacefully and with dignity" (Kessler, 1997, p. 7 f.). However, dying with dignity requires time, space and competent assistance. (DGP, 2010). These demands make it clear that a lack of structures can have a significant impact on end-of-life care.

Smith (2000, cited in Müller-Busch, 2013, p. 100 f.) lists 12 specific elements for a dignified death, which are of great importance to the people affected. These include knowing about the phenomenon of death, allowing people to die, being able to choose the place of death themselves, preserving the person's dignity and intimacy, treating pain, providing emotional support and allowing time to say goodbye. In addition, autonomy, independence and self-determination are ethical principles that are of great importance to almost all people, regardless of age. However, these norms can no longer be fully experienced in the care of others. People in need of help are particularly dependent on others and are afraid of having to spend the last days of their lives under the control of others (Engelke, 2015, p. 125).

In addition to accepting the personal life situation and respecting dignity and self-determination, it is also important to deal with the emotion of grief. This feeling manifests itself in the carer through deep consternation or emotion and gives rise to feelings of guilt, anger and rage. A bond that has been broken by death can thus become a personal loss (Stähli, 2004, p. 146). Prospective carers experience sadness when confronted with their own finiteness and in the process of saying goodbye, loss situations and separation events (Handler, 2014; Halfpap, 2009; Stähli, 2004).

Apart from grief, the feeling of fear is also a constant companion in the everyday lives of dying people. For the Italian palliative care physician G. Borasio, anxiety is sometimes the reason for the painful course of dying, as personal perception is distorted, the absorption of information is prevented and mutual communication is impossible (Borasio, 2013, p. 9 f.). Inner restlessness, depressive moods and anxiety can rarely be avoided (Riemann, 2007, cited in Engelke, 2015, p. 145).

In end-of-life care, emotions must be respected in the context of nursing tasks and these must be met with a loving attitude characterised by care and trust (Engelke, 2015, p. 145). It is always important to maintain a balance between fear and hope; only when hope is no longer there as a signpost does the dying person feel at the mercy of death (Engelke, 2015, p. 162).

2.2.3 End-of-life care in a psychosocial context

In the 1970s, Elisabeth Kübler-Ross conducted interviews with dying people and was able to demonstrate the individuality and characteristic psychosocial behaviour patterns in the dying process in over 200 interviews. Based on her observations, she defined different phases which, on the one hand, explain the reactions of the patients and, on the other, call for appropriate behaviour in care (Kränz- le, 2011, p. 18). Kübler-Ross recognised that, in addition to those affected, it is primarily the carers themselves who find it difficult to deal with dying and death and are therefore insecure and anxious (Kübler-Ross, 2013, p. 15).

However, the phase model developed should not be seen as a strict chronological model, but rather as an explanation for the behaviour of dying people in complex situations. Accordingly, end-of-life care means preserving the uniqueness of each individual person, giving hope, respecting behavioural patterns and enabling closeness through communication (Kübler-Ross, 2013, p. 13 f.). Wilkening & Kunz (2003) mention that the reactions do not always depend solely on the resident, but are also controlled by the relationship and emotional work of the carer. They thus emphasise the influence of the carer's own insecurities, fears and feelings of guilt (Wilkening & Kunz, 2003, p. 29).

In professional end-of-life care, it is therefore essential to consider the psychological and social situation of the dying person and to accept their understanding of death. It is about being touched in one's own attitude and entering into an emotional relationship with the person concerned. In everyday caring, this does not always mean giving advice in a paternalistic attitude, but rather listening and being there for the other person (Engelke, 2015, p. 88). Carers are therefore significantly involved in the experience of the dying process by looking after people until they die and involving them in decisions (Röttger, 2015). In addition to professional skills, this requires, above all, a corresponding attitude in caregiving.

2.2.4 Attitude in caring for the dying

When caring for the dying, carers are tasked daily with focussing on the person with all their needs and concerns (Ma- gon, 2014a, p. 94). Feichtner (2014, p. 15) emphasises that they are always confronted with their own finiteness and transience. In addition, they are challenged to reflect on their individual experiences and their attitude towards dying and death (Magon, 2014a, p. 94). The confrontation with the personal reality of death characterises the attitude and leads to a direct process of change (Engelke, 2015, p. 233; Kostrzewa & Kutzner, 2002, p. 38). Confronting one's own mortality also proved to be a difficulty in the qualitative study at the University Medical Centre Freiburg (2009), with only 50% of the nursing staff surveyed stating that they deal with their own mortality and are aware of their personal finiteness (Halfpap, 2009, p. 18).

Reflection, as part of the personal confrontation with dying and death, also means a confrontation with one's own transience (Feichtner, 2014, p. 15; Rest, 2006, p. 101). Reflection is therefore a prerequisite for empathic end-of-life care, which guides both behaviour and attitude in the context of care through dignity and mindfulness (Giese, 2013, p. 17; Wilkening & Kunz, 2003).

Magon (2014a, p. 94) describes one's own experiences as a "background foil of [...] experience", which guides the carers in their actions. In order not to act without reflection, a willingness to recognise the fears and needs of the dying and to become aware of values is required. Only by reflecting on and reviewing one's own attitude and experiences can ideals be corrected and shaped as a personal attitude (Augustyn, 2012, p. 18).

Behaviour as a conscious process is contrasted with attitude as a basic personal attitude. Attitude refers to a person's willingness, based on experience, to react to a person or situation in a certain judgemental way (Richard, Gero & Zimbardo, 2008). Attitude is characterised by the relationship to each other, adapted to the respective working conditions and related to the people being cared for without judging or excluding them (Hausmann & Koller, 2011, p. 186; Heller & Knipping, 2007, p. 642).

The International Council of Nurses (ICN Code, 2012) calls for attitude as an essential element in dealing with and taking responsibility for fellow human beings and those in need of care. In this context, "professional values such as respect, attentiveness and responsiveness to demands and needs, as well as compassion, trustworthiness and integrity" play an essential role in behaviour.

The Swiss Professional Association (SBK) sees attitude as respect for the ethical principles of justice, autonomy, doing good and non-harm. "Human dignity and the uniqueness of life are at the centre of nursing care" (SBK, 1990, quoted from Monteverde, 2007, p. 530). In the White Paper of the European Association for Palliative Care (EAPC), attitudes and positioning towards life and death are considered a building block of palliative care through respect for relationships, autonomy and dignity (Krumm et al., 2015, p. 156).

Attitude requires a corresponding working culture that centres on the development of trust, confidence and understanding. This enables relationships to be built, communication processes to be facilitated and the direct confrontation with dying and death to be recognised as a weakness or seen as a challenge. In addition to reflecting on one's own life, adopting a palliative attitude requires allowing, feeling and articulating farewell and grief (Heller & Knipping, 2007, p. 642 ff.).

Attitude is based on the life expressions of each individual, on the interdisciplinarity of different expertise, on the ability of all actors to reflect and on the organisation of work processes. It is about respect for personality, appreciation and respect. Wishes and feelings must be accepted, regardless of religious, cultural and ideological views (Heller & Knipping, 2007, p. 44 f.) For Pribil (2005), attitude also means "getting involved and letting go". This means that it must be possible to engage with the person themselves, their life story, experiences and emotions without preconceptions. Letting go" includes letting go of behavioural patterns and fundamental decisions, as well as emphasising individuality (Pribil, 2005, p. 185).

In connection with professional ethics, Schweidtmann (1998) carried out quantitative research among carers and doctors in the Federal Republic of Germany. On the issue of attitude, 90 % of those surveyed were convinced that safety in nursing care can be learnt by dealing with one's own attitude and the phenomenon of death and is helpful for care (Schweidtmann, 1998, p. 16 ff, cited in Griegoleit, 2011, p. 245).

In the context of care, Benner (1994) uses the term "caring" in her study "Stufen zur Pflegekompetenz", which can be equated with a caring attitude . For Benner, "caring" does not mean sacrificing oneself "but treating the other person [...] with appreciation, [...] giving commitment, inner involvement, compassion and trust". There is no room for marginalising suffering, dying and death in "caring"; on the contrary, reflecting on one's own role and accepting the illness is seen as a prerequisite (Benner, 1994, cited in Thielhorn, 2005, p. 76).

Accordingly, carers have a special task in their actions and behaviour when caring for the dying. They should create appropriate framework conditions, support the relatives and create a balance between care-related care and personal self-determination. The aim is to create conditions that make it possible to experience the last hours as worth living. Renz-Polster (2008, cited in Feichtner, 2016, p. 19) states that the experience of the last hours of life is heavily dependent on the behaviour of the carer and can be influenced by them.

Ochsmann (1993, p. 33, cited in Griegoleit, 2011, p. 124) describes avoidance behaviour when dealing with the dying. He cites the fear of an immediate encounter with death as a triggering factor for avoidance strategies and subsequent inability to act. Carers therefore enter the room of the dying person less often, avoid increased contact or deliberately spend less time with the dying person. Interestingly, the human fear of death is particularly potentiated among medical and nursing staff, which explains the avoidance of care activities, a reduction in communication and a delay in making contact with the person concerned (Feifel et al., 1967, cited in Griegoleit, 2011, p. 30).

Göckenjan (2008, p. 11) also mentioned the delay behaviour in his discussions and pointed out suppression tendencies such as time pressure or predetermined action routines. The attitude and approach of the carer therefore has a decisive influence on the behaviour of the dying person (Griegoleit, 2011, p. 130). In turn, the reduction of uncertainty and fear supports the relationship process with the patient and enables openness and truthfulness.

2.2.5 Relationship work as a challenge in counselling

Everyday nursing care is characterised by relationship work, which always takes place between two people. In the context of care, there is the patient on the one hand and the carer as a professional on the other (Bauer, 2001, p. 313). As early as the 1950s, Hildegard Peplau positioned the relationship as a central element of various nursing theories. Accordingly, care does not describe an isolated action, but a process of interaction between carer and patient (Peplau, 1997, cited in Kühne-Ponesch, 2004, pp. 127-133). The carer is part of the relationship and is connected to the person being cared for as a person in all interventions. Hildegard Peplau (1995) presents the relationship between carer and patient as a process that takes place in every comprehensive care situation in the four phases of orientation, identification, utilisation and detachment. It is a give and take, whereby carers are usually the givers first and only later the receivers (Peplau, 1995). For the psychologist Watzlawick (1990), a relationship is something growing and in flux that is experienced, lived and shaped by all those involved.

Relationship work, as part of relationship care and the content of attachment care, is understood as an active process of consciously shaping situations. Relationship care defines the shaping of relationships and has always taken place in care (Bauer, 2001, p. 311). In congruent relationship care, human affection is seen as a support and healing factor (Bauer, 2001, p. 314).

Kränzle (2011) advocates the relationship process in the care of the dying as a personal encounter in the sense of professional closeness, characterised by empathy and truthfulness. She defines this as a "temporary relationship" that will end in the foreseeable future due to death and therefore never equals the intimacy and depth of a conventional friendship (Kränzle, 2011, p. 184). For Raible (2015, p. 9), personal relationships and the offer of human closeness through touch are also of particular importance in end-of-life care, as support until the end.

For Rogers (2000, p. 22 ff., cited in Griegoleit, 2011, p. 148; Beutel, 2011, p. 37), empathy, respect, appreciation and respect for the person, as well as congruence as sincerity and authenticity in behaviour, are indispensable as part of the relationship.

Rest (2006) also believes that dignified end-of-life care is characterised by an interpersonal relationship with the dying person. This includes the principle of reciprocity, otherness and the assumption of responsibility and should be underpinned by friendly co-operation and respect (Rest, 2006, p. 168).

The "own and personal death", as it is called by Rest (2006, p. 23), serves as a hallmark of end-of-life care. This refers to assistance that is characterised by personality, space and time and one's own forms of organisation (Rest, 2006, p. 15). Rest (2006, p. 19) therefore argues in favour of a very specific term. He speaks of "caring for the dying" because this conceals the activity of the carer and focuses on accompanying and participating.

For carers, the relationship as an aspect of closeness to the patient can be a hurdle in which they must try to meet the other person competently. This is because witnessing situations and empathising with people can become a heavy burden. The difficulties therefore do not lie in the nursing skills of carers, but are often limited to the challenges of psychosocial care as part of relationship work (BGW, 2000). Müller et al. (2010, p. 229) were also able to prove that the relationship with the dying person is a stress factor, whereby closeness is also mentioned here as positive, but at the same time is often perceived as stressful. In addition to Müller et al. (2010), Halfpap (2009, p. 15) also emphasises the existence of an emotional bond and the inability to set boundaries as a psychological stress factor. As a result, it can be assumed that the encounter with dying and death, due to socialisation experiences and structural circumstances, represents a considerable stress factor for professional carers, but especially for prospective carers. In the course of this work, various aspects that need to be considered by carers when providing professional end-of-life care will be explained in more detail.

2.3 Dying and death in long-term inpatient care

The care of people at the end of their lives is increasingly becoming a central task for residential care facilities for the elderly. These facilities are particularly challenged as places of death.

Inpatient long-term care facilities provide round-the-clock catering and care for people in need of care (Rest, 2006, p. 73; National Ethics Council, 2006, p. 41). Accommodation in retirement and nursing homes becomes the centre of life and place of residence for the last years of life, right up to the place of death for the person concerned (DGP, 2012). The institutions offer people a "last home" when living in their own home is no longer possible (Giese, 2013, p. 14). The term "need for care" is defined by a physical or psychological condition that lasts for at least six months. The person concerned is dependent on the help of others for personal hygiene, nutrition and mobilisation (Wilkening & Kunz, 2003, p. 16).

2.3.1 Retirement and nursing homes as places of death

After hospitals, care facilities are the second most common place to say goodbye and die for around 30% of people (Seeger, 2011, p. 164). According to Statistics Austria (2014), 17.44% of the 78,252 deaths in Austria occurred in care and nursing homes. In Germany, a figure of 25 - 30 % is given (Engel- ke, 2015, p. 47). Dasch et al. (2015) conducted a population-based study in Germany (Westphalia Lippe region) on the issue of current places of death, in which they compared the places of death over a decade, from 2001 to 2011. The study showed that the hospital is the most common place of death, accounting for 51.2 % of deaths. This was followed by the home environment with 23.0% and retirement and nursing homes with 19.0%. However, retirement and nursing homes recorded the sharpest increase as a place of death at 6.8% (Dasch et al., 2015, p. 498).

Admission to a nursing home takes place either directly from hospital or from home and can therefore be unplanned and unprepared (En- gelke, 2015, p. 213; DGP, 2012). The fact that retirement and nursing homes are increasingly becoming places of death is also due to the high admission age and increasingly short length of stay of residents and the lack of social support networks (DGP, 2012). In addition, the chronic illnesses of residents do not lead directly to death, but are very complex and require appropriate symptom control and support in the final phase. Borasio, one of Europe's leading palliative physicians, emphasises that for many people, dying in a nursing home is perceived as very terrible and frightening (Borasio, 2012, p. 34).

These facilities play a central role in the care of elderly and dying people and are therefore faced with the challenge of providing dignified care for very elderly, dying people in their last phase of life (Heller, 2007). People are moving into care homes later and later, and those who are often already in great need of care die very soon after being admitted (Gerhard, 2015, p. 197; Seeger, 2011, p. 165). According to the National Ethics Council (2006, p. 41), 30% of people die within the first three months. Inpatient long-term care facilities are therefore places of care where death is omnipresent and the last weeks or, at best, years of life are spent (Seeger, 2011, p. 164). The German Society for Palliative Medicine therefore calls for inpatient care facilities to develop into " [...] places for liveable ageing and dignified dying" and to recognise dying as a natural process (DGP, 2012).

2.3.2 Reasons for increasing institutionalisation

Increased life expectancy and the increasing individualisation of lifestyles have changed the way in which dying people are treated and placed death in institutions designed for this purpose. The fear of isolation and loneliness are at the centre of this (Röttger, 2015).

At the same time, the conditions for dying with dignity in institutions are not always or only inadequately provided due to organisational structures. Regardless of this, Engelke (2015) poses the question of whether the cause is not the lack of willingness on the part of society to accompany elderly and terminally ill people. Care in inpatient long-term care facilities relieves the social and family environment of its responsibility and at the same time makes it easier to criticise existing deficits and inadequacies (Engelke, 2015, p. 29).

As a result, the care of the dying is increasingly left to professional carers and disappears from everyday life and the social environment (Jenull et al., 2006). Rest (2006, p. 172) even attests to a tendency to exclude the dying from social society. The Bioethics Commission of the Austrian Federal Chancellery (2015) states that this professionalism and expertise is not only assumed but also expected by society. The care of those people who need help and support is thus increasingly seen as a social responsibility and attributed to organisations and professions (Engelke, 2015, p. 54). The reasons cited for this are the unwillingness of relatives to take on the care, spatial conditions at home, personal attitudes or family situations (Engelke, 2015, p. 49 ff.). The Bioethics Commission (2015) cites changing living conditions and family structures as well as insufficient social networks in old age as further reasons.

Residents of care homes feel this development and perceive social isolation. Engelke (2015, p. 212) is very critical of this fact and expresses his concerns in this regard. For him, people in retirement and care homes are even "at the mercy of freezing and dying". In this context, the death researcher pleads for the support of relatives and loved ones, with whose cooperation a social participation in life and corresponding assistance is possible (Engelke, 2015, p. 216).

Due to the fact of institutionalisation and the need for dignified and humane support, Wilkening & Kunz (2003,

p. 84) call for a corresponding work and farewell culture in retirement and nursing homes. The "culture of living and dying" represents a system of values, norms and attitudes and accepts dying as a natural process (Wilkening & Kunz, 2003, p. 17).

2.3.3 Farewell culture in residential care homes for the elderly

Engelke (2015, p. 43) and Heller & Wegleitner (2011, p. 73) also point out that care homes have increasingly developed into "homes for the dying". This makes the demand for palliative care with an appropriate attitude all the more understandable. Especially when the end of life is approaching, consideration of the physical, mental and social dimensions, supported by a holistic care philosophy, is essential as a culture of dying (Wilkening & Kunz, 2003, p. 31).

Open discussion through empathic dialogue and interaction should be a concern for all those involved in the process. Residents must be involved in decision-making and supported in their individual quality of life. The care concept of activating care, which is applied in these facilities, can certainly be supplemented with palliative aspects and practised as an interdisciplinary team approach (Wilkening & Kunz, 2003, p. 108 ff.).

Wilkening & Kunz (2003) emphasise a person-centred, needs-oriented approach to seriously ill and dying people. "You don't have to do things any longer, you have to do them differently." (Wilkening & Kunz, 2003, p. 221). These aspects should be discussed in training and demanded in everyday nursing care. Those affected often only want to experience the complete takeover of care in the terminal phase, until then they want to be as independent as possible (Engelke, 2015, p. 128).

Falkenstein (2001, p. 165) was able to prove that for more than two thirds of the carers surveyed, it is not possible to care for the dying in an old people's and nursing home in the way that they personally consider to be right and that their professional self-image demands. Carers often have a different idea of end-of-life care, but are not always able to implement it. Due to the lack of organisational guidelines, end-of-life care therefore takes place very individually and differently. Pleschberger (2005, p. 69) points out that the quality of end-of-life care depends not only on personal attitudes, but above all on the qualifications of the carers.

Even though retirement and nursing homes play a central role in the care of dying people, the question arises as to what importance is actually attached to or understood by end-of-life care in these institutions. The demand for the involvement of carers in the sense of palliative care places high demands, as outlined below.

2.3.4 Palliative care in the elderly care setting

Holistic care enables elderly and seriously ill people to shape their final phase of life in a self-determined way and thus to die with dignity. Palliative geriatrics, as a sub-area of palliative care, represents a "common intersection of geriatrics and palliative medicine" and prioritises the preservation of quality of life as the highest objective (Kunz & Wilkening, 2003, p. 82 ff.). Multimorbid, elderly people with several age-related, chronic illnesses are at the centre of nursing care.

The focus of all interactions is on the person and their needs, as well as respect for their activity and acceptance of self-determination (Steffen & Bürgi, 2011, p. 32). Müller-Busch (2014, p. 1) emphasises needs-oriented care, particularly for the elderly, and underlines "[...] empathetic end-of-life care and effective communication while respecting the needs and wishes of the person concerned."

Individual symptoms are often difficult to attribute to a specific illness due to their complexity (Gerhard, 2015, p. 197). In the terminal phase, the focus is therefore on needs- and resident-orientated care (Kunz & Wilkening, 2003, p. 84 f.). In this phase, Kunz & Wilkening (2003, p. 87) call for conventional care measures to no longer be routinely applied, for automated work processes to be avoided and for resident-orientated action to be taken.

Rest (2006, p. 73) attests not only to the awareness of complexity among older people, but also to the fact that death must not be seen as a failure or failure in inpatient long-term care facilities, but rather as a natural phenomenon of life. In addition to this, Giese (2013, p. 15) calls for a special "protected space for the dying" in the retirement and nursing home setting, where the resident is withdrawn from daily routine treatments and human dying is made possible. For Pleschberger (2003, cited in Knipping, 2007, p. 132), "respect and preservation of dignity" plays a central role in the development of this attitude and culture, especially in the nursing home institution.

The Charter for the Care of the Seriously Ill and Dying in Germany calls for the implementation of palliative treatment concepts and the development of a hospice culture, particularly in inpatient care structures (DGP, 2010). The policy paper on the development of "Hospice culture and palliative care in inpatient care facilities for the elderly" therefore specifies concrete implementation strategies that take into account the needs of people with multiple chronic illnesses and are intended to make dying worth living (DGP, 2012).

Despite the fact that end-of-life care plays a central role in the everyday life of inpatient long-term care facilities, the question arises as to how this is dealt with in everyday life.

2.3.5 Stress factors for carers

In order to describe the stress factors, it is essential to reflect on the organisational self-image of the respective institution on the one hand and the professional self-image of the carers on the other (Griegoleit, 2011, p. 26).

The aim of a study carried out by Koch-Straube (1997) on the perception of the living and working environment of nursing homes was to ascertain the concerns and burdens of carers with regard to care concepts, work with relatives, framework conditions, etc. In the context of end-of-life care, it was shown that the employees experience "the encounter with serious illnesses and dying as a situation of extreme helplessness and lack of success". Above all, being alone with dying people and the demand for possible decisions represent a great challenge. Their own expectations of holistic care often diverge from the reality of functional care, which is expressed in the care of the dying with excessive demands and helplessness (Koch-Straube, 1997, p. 9).

George (2014) currently analyses the dying situation at nursing, medical and psychosocial level in German inpatient care facilities. In a quantitative survey of 467 institutions (n = 2,613)

were asked about personnel and institutional resources for training, working atmosphere, communication, symptom control, life support, education and stress factors. The structural conditions in the facilities were rated as satisfactory and better than expected. The number of residents who have to die without the presence of relatives or carers is perceived as problematic and stressful. An equally problematic stress situation is the time and personnel resources available. Only 34% of the carers surveyed reported that they were able to provide optimal end-of-life care, although 75% of carers would be able to provide dignified care in the last days of life in a nursing home if the right conditions were in place (George, 2014).

From 1999 to 2004, the Centre for Work and Organisational Research conducted a study on "End-of-life care in Saxony" among 4,200 people in the Federal Republic of Germany (BGW, 2000). The influences of privacy, premises, human attention and pain therapy were named, with the factor of lack of time representing the highest stress factor. More than 50 % of the professional groups surveyed stated that dealing with and caring for the dying is very demanding. Younger carers in particular (< 35 years) feel very insecure and helpless when providing care. Older carers (> 45 years), on the other hand, complain of overload and conflicts with relatives and loved ones. This confirms the assumption that increasing professional experience correlates with less stress. The level of stress is the same, only the feeling of powerlessness and helplessness as well as fear of failure is even more pronounced in younger carers (BGW, 2000).

In addition to Koch-Straube (1997) and George (2014), Wilkening & Kunz (2003) also cite specific stress factors in the context of caring for the dying. On the one hand, extrinsic stress factors include an insufficient focus on dying and death as part of training. On the other hand, the authors point to an insensitive approach to the first death in practice and cite a lack of framework conditions for dignified end-of-life care as factors of disappointment. In addition to time pressure, inadequate interest and motivation as well as a lack of emotional competence are also cited (Wilkening & Kunze, 2003, p. 139).

The performance of activating care activities is cited as an intrinsic stress factor. This is related to the fact that the use of needs-orientated support is required but not always carried out. The mediating role in working with relatives, the verbal, derogatory tone with the dying person, the confrontation with fear and pain, as well as the refusal of food and fluids are experienced as stressful care-related factors (Wilkening & Kunze, 2003, p. 140 f.). Food and fluid intake is also a stress factor for Werner (2013), especially when it comes to refusing food and drink. Carers describe helplessness in their actions and uncertainty in possible decision-making issues (Werner, 2013, p. 30).

In the context of intrinsic stress, May (1999, cited in Pleschberger 2005, p. 67) states that carers actually spend most of their time assisting the dying with basic care, such as administering food or assisting with excretion, and consequently invest less time in psychosocial support. The reasons for this are not denounced.

However, whether carers react by reducing contact depends on their awareness of the expectation of death, i.e. the time and certainty of death. However, this is linked to a certain expectation. If, for example, there is no hoped-for improvement in the patient's condition, carers reduce their involvement and the frequency of care sequences (Griegoleit, 2011, p. 98 f.). The reason for this is seen on the one hand in socialisation and the teaching of certain norms, and on the other hand in the emphasis on the somatic and neglect of the emotional level during training. In addition, Griegoleit (2011, p. 100) observes the process organisation and structure and Halfpap (2009) the spatial and temporal conditions of the respective organisation as a stress factor. As a result, there is a marginal needs assessment of the needs and wishes of affected residents in need of assistance.

In the course of this work, the fears and needs that are specifically observed in elderly and very elderly dying people and that can be a challenge for carers are identified.

2.3.6 Needs as a challenge in caring

More and more people want a "humane death" that is characterised by humanity, personality and self-determination (Rest, 2006, p. 200). In a current statement by the Bioethics Commission (2015), it is pointed out that the needs, wishes and problems in all dimensions must also be recognised, taken into account and fulfilled.

Encounters with dying and death inevitably take on concrete forms in old age, through the death of peers, a partner, the accompaniment of relatives or the beginning of one's own dying process. Nevertheless, elderly people in need of care have different ideas about death, depending on their emotional, psychological or mental state. Under no circumstances should these be negated due to carers' fears. Dying and death must be addressed openly and the discussion must not be taken for granted (Wilkening & Kunz, 2003, p. 22 f.).

For the National Ethics Council (2006, p. 47), in addition to coping with physical demands, recognising psychosocial needs also plays a role. Moreover, an increasing need for help and care leads to a loss of self-determination and quality of life. To counteract this development, the following three aspects must be ensured in complex care situations. These are relationship building and the conscious perception of needs, empathic communication and emotional support, as well as comprehensive counselling and information on the resident's condition and possible decision-making (Wasner, 2013, p. 11 f.). A study carried out at the University Hospital of Cologne in 2009 shows that needs can be assessed primarily through dialogue. In the study, psychosocial well-being, self-determination and emotional support were also recorded as concrete wishes (Vogt, 2010).

Heimerl et al. (2000, cited in Heimerl, 2007, p. 134) were able to identify the following needs of older people on the basis of qualitative interviews, which also coincide with the statements by Magon (2014a, p. 155). This is the desire not to have to suffer and not to be in pain. It is also important for people to receive appropriate information about their state of health. In addition, the need for shared endurance and involvement in decision-making through co-determination is at the centre of this. Residents of long-term care facilities primarily offer the desire for companionship so that they do not have to die alone (Magon, 2014b, p. 155; Heimerl, 2002, cited in Heimerl, 2007, p. 134 f.). Müller-Busch (2013, p. 103) also sees autonomy as the ability to take responsibility, make decisions and realise oneself as a "basic element [...] of human life". Only through self-determination can the dying realise their own identity and feel human (Müller-Busch, 2013, p. 104). In addition to the need for information and autonomy, Kränzle (2011, p. 20) and Borasio (2012, p. 60) emphasise above all the need for multi-professional, open communication between the carer and the dying person.

An international review by Davies & Higginson (2008) shows the specific needs of older and very old people. However, the authors also point out deficits in care, especially symptom control. In order to ensure assistance in dying, an appropriate work culture, supportive organisational conditions, time resources and reflection on routine treatments are required (Engelke, 2015, p. 213 f.; Seeger, 2011, p. 165).

The German policy paper on the development of "Hospice culture and palliative care in inpatient facilities for the elderly" therefore claims that the organisation must shape the working culture in such a way "that the person in need and not the functional processes are in the foreground" (DGP, 2012, p. 21).

After mentioning the treatment of the dying in retirement and nursing homes, the following chapter will look specifically at the perspective of trainees.

2.4 Dying and death in nursing training

Personal support and cross-institutional care for the dying will become increasingly important because end-of-life care does not take place in individual, specialised facilities, but must be implemented everywhere (Pleschberger & Heimerl, 2005, p. 15).

This makes the confrontation with dying and death, especially during training, all the more emotionally and psychologically demanding, the mastery of which cannot be taken for granted (Widegger et al., 2011).

The state of research on dealing with dying and death from the perspective of nursing students is presented below. After citing the legal framework conditions, the term "death education" is defined and specific stress factors and fears in the context of end-of-life care are listed.

2.4.1 Legal framework conditions in the training programme

In the 1997 amendment to the Healthcare and Nursing Act, the mandatory implementation of the subject "palliative care" in the training regulations took account of the establishment of palliative care in the context of training (GuKG, 1997, cited in Ple- schberger & Heimerl, 2005, p. 16; GuK-AV, 1999).

In addition to the further development of job profiles, the 2016 amendment to the GuKG also introduced new competences and areas of activity for the nursing assistant professions and the higher-level service. As in other European countries, training to become a senior healthcare and nursing professional now takes place in the tertiary education sector and is based at universities of applied sciences. The one-year training programme to become a nursing assistant and the two-year training programme to become a specialist nursing assistant is provided in schools for healthcare and nursing. The dual training system will be retained up to this point (Weiss & Lust, 2017).

In the future, generalist training programme for the advanced level of healthcare and nursing, a reduction in teaching in the subject of palliative care to up to less than a third is being considered, although the curriculum is still in the design phase and therefore no specific details are available. However, given the number of hours required, it will be difficult for teachers to raise awareness of dying and death through appropriate discussion as part of death education (Kössler, 2016, p. 8).

2.4.2 Dying and death in an educational context

Death education or thanatogogy refers to the teaching of how to deal with dying and death as a processual discussion in an educational context (Petzold, 1965, cited in Griegoleit, 2011, p. 133). In Austria and Germany, methodological implementation began at the end of the 1980s in the form of seminars for doctors and carers. The aim was to prepare the professional groups mentioned for dealing with the dying and to carry out their own reflection work (Griegoleit, 2011, p.137). In a study on the current stressful situations in end-of-life care, carers still state that there is insufficient preparation for end-of-life care as part of basic training, although this has been part of the curriculum since 1997 (BGM, 2000).

Wittowski (2012, p. 65, cited in Maywald, 2014) names the following aspects that should be achieved through death ecudation in teaching. Prioritising the learning of openness in order to be able to talk about the topic of dying (Maywald, 2014, p. 35; Ek et al., 2014). In order to develop this ability, Heimerl & Pleschberger (2005, p. 23) call for an examination of dying and death on the one hand and confrontation with death during practical training on the other, which of course cannot be guaranteed.

In addition, it is important for the practical instructors to clarify uncertainties and address stresses and strains at the practical training centre and for the teachers at the school (Kunz, 2007, p. 52). Personal or family experience in caring for the dying must not be taken for granted, but must be learnt and reflected upon. Terry and Carroll (2008) report in the context of accompanying trainees that they repeatedly feel left alone and inadequately accompanied. Halfpap (2009, p. 22) can also confirm the lack of psychological support: in the study conducted in Germany, almost 25% of the nursing students surveyed stated that they were left alone during mentoring. Beatty (2013, p. 20) adds that the mentoring of nursing students "[...] tends to be left to chance". The resulting uncertainty has an impact on communication behaviour and may even be responsible for students dropping out of training. Schmidt (2010, p. 643) therefore argues in favour of "sensitive and understanding support and guidance", which can only be ensured through an open approach and consideration of personal influencing factors.

2.4.3 Influence of experiential knowledge in the experience of care

Caring for the dying is a challenge for society as a whole, but is part of the professional field of activity and role model of professional carers (Heimerl & Pleschberger, 2005, p. 25 ff.). Carers occupy a special position, but are challenged both emotionally and psychologically (Charalambous & Kaite, 2013).

For trainees who come into contact with dying and death for the first time, accompanying the dying means a sudden, often even abrupt confrontation with their own finiteness (Feichtner, 2014, p. 15). Although death is omnipresent today, it is not real, but fictionalised in the media and in people's own imaginations (Student et al., 2004). In addition to the lack of personal experience, both Pinho & Barbosa (2010) and Borsio (2012, p. 29 f.) state that due to increasing institutionalisation, young people hardly have any personal contact with the dying. Contact and interaction with the dying is becoming a rarity in young people's lives. Trainees often only come into contact with dying and death during their work placement and therefore report a lack of experiences of loss (Widegger et al., 2011; Parry, 2011). Due to their lack of experience, they are therefore also referred to as "laypeople in dealing with dying and death" (Schmidt, 2010, p. 642). Heimerl & Pleschberger (2005, p. 23) add to this a marginal discussion and increasing taboo in everyday care practice. However, as the carers themselves are often overwhelmed by the situation, the trainees cannot demand their support and are left to their own devices (Pinho & Barbosa, 2010).

These findings are consistent with the research conducted by Halbmayr-Kubicsek (2015) on Austrian bachelor's degree students in healthcare and nursing. If they already have personal experience of dealing with the dying before their first placement, they have fewer fears and anxieties. Ohlrogge (2012) also found that students benefit from private experiences in the family environment, whereas death is frightening without previous experience. Experience in confronting the dying therefore facilitates an open approach (Andraschko, 2008, p. 13).

To summarise, it can be said that when confronted with dying and death, one's own experiences play an essential role in one's personal attitude and emotional processing in order to be able to cope with the situations listed below.

2.4.4 Selected stress factors for the trainees

With regard to personal stress factors, the main stress factors in caring for the dying are ignorance in dealing with the dying, helplessness in acting, uncertainty in supporting relatives, carrying out care measures and access to closeness and distance. However, it should be noted that trainees also have a certain curiosity and face the situation with open expectations (Halbmayr-Kubicsek, 2015, p. 599 f.). Heimerl & Pleschberger (2005, p. 25 ff.) cite proximity to the dying person, dealing with pain and distressing symptoms, caring for relatives and collaboration with other professional groups as challenging factors in end-of-life care.

In addition to psychosocial aspects, Albrecht (2010, p. 523) describes above all physical conditions such as physical weakness, nausea, chronic pain, changes in consciousness

pain, changes in consciousness, refusal of food and fluids and raspy breathing as stressful factors. The demand for physical touch or the rejection of closeness and communication can create feelings of insecurity and powerlessness (Pribil, 2005, p. 195 ff.). However, Ohlrogge (2012) points out that it is not the individual symptoms that have an aggravating effect, but rather the complexity of a situation that is stressful. Beatty (2013, p. 7) and Widegger et al. (2011, p. 108) also describe the duration and intensity of care as demanding. In the studies by Müller et al. (2010), the relationship is also named as the second most common stress factor (Müller, Pfister, Markett & Jaspers, 2010, p. 229). The aspect of the relationship, characterised by closeness and contact, is at the centre of nursing activities, particularly in long-term care facilities, and shows the emotional effects listed below.

2.4.5 Emotional reactions during care

Dealing with suffering and fear of death is a new challenge and is usually accompanied by emotional demands and distress (Terry & Caroll, 2008). The trainees are strongly guided by their personal feelings. These subsequently influence the individual steps they take and their actions (Handler, 2013; Ohlrogge, 2012; Andrasch- ko, 2008).

Unknown emotions such as anxiety, excessive demands or self-doubt can be triggered (Beatty, 2013; Widegger et al., 2013). Other feelings described include personal dismay, helplessness, anger, aggression, powerlessness, sadness, shock, disgust and shame (Ohlrog- ge, 2012; Müller et al., 2010; Stähli, 2004). In addition, Handler (2014) also cites joy, gratitude, friendliness and affection as positive emotions. In her work, the author was able to show that younger carers in particular experience positive emotions (Handler, 2014, p. 219). In Ohlrogge's (2012) study, trainees report a feeling of satisfaction, but only when care is possible.

Widegger, Schulc & Them (2011) make clear reference to emotional dissonance (Widegger et al., 2011, cited in Handler, 2014, p. 212). This term refers to the difference between what a carer feels in a situation and what they should or may feel. The question arises as to whether the feelings should fit in with the generally applicable norms or whether the behaviour should be changed according to the feelings (Widegger et al., 2011, p. 103). The results of a study by Kersting (2005) confirm that trainees often act intuitively, i.e. according to their feelings. Their behaviour in action is shaped and influenced by the organisation and structure.

In the context of end-of-life care, Rest (2006) even describes the unprepared assumption of care for the dying by trainees as "criminal". Before the first encounter, he calls for preparation through appropriate action-orientated learning methods and opportunities for discussion during training by trusted persons (Rest, 2006, p. 274). Grie- goleit (2011, p. 9) emphasises that emotional processing or open communication must be given space for end-of-life care.

CHAPTER 3

Empirical part

Interview research using a qualitative research design was chosen to conduct the empirical study. The aim is to consider the personal experiences of dealing with dying and death as a context-bound subject to be researched and to explore these in the context of nursing training (Mayer, 2007, p. 87).

3.1 Research design

The qualitative research approach is justified by the object of investigation. This approach of phenomenology, as a direction of qualitative research, is rooted in philosophy and goes back to the work of Husserl, Heidegger and Gadamer. The aim is to understand experiences and events and to explore their relevance for the individual (Mayer, 2007, p. 91).

In qualitative research, a phenomenon is explored from the perspective of those affected and analysed in relation to the subject matter. This allows different approaches to the topic to be explained and conclusions to be drawn about the phenomenon under investigation (Flick, 2012, p. 95 f.). Social, often complex facts are subjectively collected, verbally transmitted, interpreted and generalised (Gläser & Laudel, 2010, p. 27). Flick (2012) further describes the appropriateness of the research object to the method, the consideration and analysis of diverse perspectives, the construction of reality and social backgrounds as well as the reflection of the researcher as essential core points of qualitative research (Flick, 2012, p. 97).

In addition, the generalisation process through induction, the focus on the subject through problem orientation, description through

openness and interpretation through pre-understanding are also seen as "pillars of qualitative thinking" (Mayer, 2002, p. 26). The results are not numerical figures, but descriptions of the interviewee (Mayer, 2007, p. 87). In order to be able to verify this claim of qualitative thought processes, the following defined criteria are required.

3.1.1 Criteria of qualitative research

In qualitative research design, the classic quality criteria of objectivity, validity, reliability and verifiability are considered critical due to subjectivity and possible differences in interpretation (Mayring, 2010, p. 116). For qualitative research, Steinke (2000) cites communicative validation as the evaluation of the data by the group of people being researched, triangulation as the use of several methods, validation as the objective examination of the interview situation and authenticity as the appropriateness in dealing with the people being analysed (Steinke, 2000, p. 321).

In this work, the criteria of consistent procedural documentation, argumentative interpretation validation, rule-guidedness, proximity to the object and object appropriateness are operationalised. Communicative validation and triangulation are not included (Mayring, 2002, p. 147).

3.1.2 Ethical premises

Within the research process, the "three basic ethical principles of privacy protection" must be observed. These include information, voluntary participation, anonymity and the protection of the individual (Mayer, 2007, p. 62). The Belmont Report, which cites the principles of respect for human dignity, beneficence and justice, can also be used as an ethical guideline here (DGP, n.d.).

The ethical premises were taken into account in this study by informing the subjects in accordance with the principle of voluntary informed consent and the anonymous analysis of the data collected by the researcher herself (Flick, 2012, p. 64; Gläser & Laudel, 2010, p. 50 f.). The interviewees signed an information sheet in which they were made aware of the right to anonymity, the confidential handling of the data and the possibility of cancelling their participation (Appendix 5). They were informed in the interview consent form that their statements would have no effect on their theoretical or practical training (Appendix 4). The data collection took place during working or school hours on the premises of the Bad Ischl, Gmunden and Vöcklabruck health and nursing schools. When scheduling the interviews, the respondents' wishes were taken into account. The students were not to incur any additional time or organisational costs (Gläser & Laudel, 2010, p. 51).

3.2 Research process

In a qualitative research process, verifiability is not the top priority due to the limited standardisability. For intersubjective comprehensibility, the documentation of the research process, the interpretation of the groups with existing data and the application of codified procedures must be ensured. This involves documenting data collection and evaluation methods, transcription rules, collected data and the process of individual decisions (Steinke, 2000, p.

326).

3.2.1 Selection of the sample

The research study was conducted at the training institutions of the Salzkammergutklinikum in Upper Austria with the locations Bad Ischl, Gmunden and Vöcklabruck. At the time of the survey (January to August 2017), a total of 242 students were completing their training, 101 of them in Gmunden (GM), 75 students in Vöcklabruck (VB) and 66 students at the Bad Ischl (BI) site.

Sampling in qualitative research must fulfil the criteria of usefulness and appropriateness in order to be able to collect and describe the desired information. The aim was to achieve a sample size of at least 15 pupils.

Twenty pupils (n = 20) from the second and third year of training were selected to carry out the research. The acquisition and information about the study was carried out by the respective heads of class at the nursing schools. The choice of sampling was voluntary and for a specific purpose. The criteria for selecting the sample was a completed internship in the extramural sector. In addition, contact and participation in accompanying dying residents for at least two days was a prerequisite. Negative experiences, age and the frequency of accompaniment were not used as criteria for participation.

3.2.2 Preparation and collection of data

The focussed, semi-structured interview, which was conducted face to face, served as the method for data collection (Gläser & Laudel, 2010, p. 41 ff.). The instrument is characterised by the use of an interview guide with semi-structured questions (Moser, 2012, p. 92). The advantage of an interview over other qualitative survey methods lies in the focussing of relevant facts. This allows precisely determinable information to be collected that emerges from actions, attitudes and personal understanding (Gläser & Laudel, 2010, p. 40).

The questions should not be seen as binding and can be changed during the interview (Gläser & Laudel, 2010, p. 42). The quality criteria of specificity, depth and person-centredness apply, in which the people should be motivated to make personal statements through follow-up questions (Lamnek, 2010, p. 338).

In order to achieve a qualitative design for the interview guide in line with the criteria listed, a written survey was conducted in advance with a total of eight nursing students (n = 8) from all training years (Appendix 1). The trainees listed their experiences of dealing with dying and death as part of their work placement in a retirement and nursing home. The survey was open-ended, with the option of three sub-questions to support the trainees' thoughts. The texts were then analysed by the researcher colour-coding frequently occurring text passages. These were then summarised in umbrella terms, condensed into main topics and used as the basis for the conception of the topic areas in the interview guide.

Before the trial interviews were conducted, the guidelines were validated by two independent nursing educators. Three interviews were then conducted, analysed and the questions in the guideline evaluated accordingly.

Gläser & Laudel (2010) recommend adapting the content of the questions to the individual subject areas when constructing the guidelines (Gläser & Laudel, 2010, p. 142). This provides orientation and enables a comparable structure in the interview.

Subjective views can be recorded promptly and presented in a comprehensible manner (Flick, 2012, p. 195; Lamnek, 2010, p. 337). A logical sequence is followed, from simple to complex content, from impersonal to personal context and from situational description to personal statement (Stigler & Felbinger, 2005, p. 129 ff.) (Appendix 2, 3). The aspects of non-influence, specificity and situational definition described by Flick (2012) can be ensured through unstructured, open questions as well as a non-judgemental statement and restraint on the part of the interviewer. Understanding of a broad spectrum can be achieved by expressing all views relevant to the interviewee. This also means that new points of view not mentioned in the guideline are addressed, provided they are important to the interviewee and do not deviate from the topic. Profundity and a personal frame of reference are provided by addressing emotional reactions and focussing on feelings (Flick, 2012, p. 195 ff.).

The pupils were therefore encouraged to speak in dialect in order to express their feelings authentically and report their experiences as congruently as possible. The requirement to speak High German could possibly lead to irritation among those affected and thus to a distorted and inadequate statement.

A total of 19 (n = 19) interviews could be analysed; only one interview (B14) proved to be unusable, as the trainee described her experiences as a geriatric care worker and not as a student.

3.2.3 Analysing and evaluating the data

In qualitative research, the data obtained is analysed using interpretative methods, which describe, explain and explicate a complex, subjective situation (Gläser & Laudel, 2010, p. 27). The interviews were transcribed by the researcher herself using the transcription software F4plus in order to prepare the data for analysis. Since the focus of this work was on the thematic content, the transcription was carried out in standardised written German by standardising the grammatical language form in order to clarify the overall picture. Notational forms of non-linguistic expressions or parts of communication were deliberately omitted. Non-verbal and emotional expressions were noted in the interview guide as verbal protocols (Mayer, 2007, p. 238; Mayring, 2002,

p. 91).

To analyse the text material, content structuring was used as a deductive category application in an interpretative reductive procedure (Mayring, 2010, p. 92). Structured content analysis is suitable because the formation of categories allows several aspects of the topic complex to be analysed, which were addressed in different contexts (Mayring, 2002, p. 118).

Interpretative-reductive methods in a qualitative analysis are descriptive and remain with the definitive content without looking for meanings in the analysis (Mayer, 2007, p. 242). With the method of qualitative content analysis, linguistic data material is selected through reduction, compared and systematised in the explication and then processed through theory-led construction (Mayring, 2002, p. 114). The coding was carried out by recognising key passages and subsequently combining them into the individual categories (Mayer, 2007, p. 244).

3.2.4 Methodology of qualitative data analysis

By transparently describing the individual steps in the research process, the content analysis procedure can be understood and the interpretation communicated in an argumentative manner (Gläser & Laudel, 2010, p. 206). This fulfils the criteria of reliability, verifiability and stringency in qualitative research processes (Holloway & Wheeler, 1996, p. 202).

Qualitative content analysis enables a systematic, rule-based text analysis of processes through systematised and verifiable analysis steps of the interpretations. For this purpose, the individual steps are analysed in detail and the results are evaluated in a controlled manner (Mayring, 2002, p. 114). In addition to summarisation and explication, structuring is the third technique of qualitative content analysis. The form of content structuring filters out certain aspects from the collected data material and summarises it in theoretically based categories (Mayring, 2010, p. 94).

At the heart of structured content analysis is the use of categories, which, by operationalising terms, are intended to ensure comprehensibility, intersubjective verifiability and comparability through the systematic data analysis and serve to structure the text material. The research process is thus made accessible, verifiable and plausible for outsiders (Mayring, 2010, p. 48 ff.).

In a deductive category application, the code system is derived from the questions, theoretically based evaluation points are applied to the data material and assigned to the text passages. The development of the category system and the course of the analysis are modelled in a continuous revision and review of the research question and data material (Mayring, 2010, p. 60). No data is lost through the formation of further subcategories, but is systematically analysed and made comprehensible in its completeness (Mayring, 2010, p. 49).

Subjectivity in the categorisation of text passages (coding) was counteracted by defining the categories and creating anchor examples and coding rules. The anchor examples as prototypical formulations were listed as memo codes and comments in the MAXQDA data analysis programme. In the computer-aided analysis, it is possible to count the codes quantitatively and compare them with other codes, which was also utilised by the researcher (Moser, 2012).

A coding guide was created for the exact allocation of the individual text modules and the code allocation (Mayring, 2010, p. 92). However, for organisational and time reasons, it was not possible to check the intercoder reliability by means of a further interrating and the analysis of several researchers within the scope of this study.

3.2.5 Procedure of the analysis

Mayring (2002) describes a three-step procedure for systematically determining whether a text component belongs to a category. By defining the categories, it is determined which parts of the material belong to a common category. Anchor examples serve as support by selecting and specifying concrete passages from the transcript. Coding rules are established to ensure correct categorisation. Text passages are colour-coded and structured. After a first pass of the review, the categories are reconsidered and categorisations are reduced or redefined. The existing category system is revised in further material runs (Mayring, 2002, p. 120).

In this study, the material was first analysed manually and then computer-assisted three times. In the manual evaluation, all text passages were read several times in a printed form using the method of initiating text work, central terms were marked and colour-coded (Kuckartz, 2016, p. 56). The focus was on familiarising themselves with the material and recognising key passages. During this initial analysis process, thoughts from statements were recorded in writing as memos and the main codes were formed deductively or a priori (Kuckartz, 2016, p. 64).

In a further step, the main categories were developed and assigned, which were derived from the main themes of the interviews. This was followed by the inductive formation of the subcategories in the second material run. The next step in the coding process involved the complete categorisation of all the data material. In a further step, these were checked for suitability and partially re-categorised (Kuckartz, 2016, p. 100).

The assignment and categorisation was carried out using QDA software and was performed in the MAXQDA12 database program.

Structured content analysis according to Mayring (2002) was used to process the data. The implementation corresponds to the flow chart listed and is based on the model of Gläser & Laudel (2010, p. 203) and Kuckartz (2012, p. 100). The process was recorded in the research diary.

CHAPTER 4

Results

The data analyses resulted in a collection of 432 codes. The text material was structured into four main categories of experience and influencing factors and subsequently assigned to a further 21 subcategories. The structure is shown in Figure 2. The number of codes reflects the frequency of the respective segments and quantitatively shows particularly relevant aspects.Figure 1: Illustration of main and sub-categories (own illustration)

Main category	*Subcategory 1*	*Subcategory 2*	*Number of Code*
A *Experience in the role as a trainee*	A 1 Understanding of role		25
	A 2 Expectations		30
	A 3 Effects on everyday working life		14
	A 4 Support from carers		36
	A 5 Theory-practice transfer		9
B *Emotions in experience*	B 1 Type of emotions		40
		B 1/1 Relieving emotions	22
		B 1/2 Stressful emotions	18
	B 2 Triggers for emotions		41
	B 3 Dealing with emotions		15
C *Person-related influencing factors*	C 1 Experience		23
	C 2 Attitude and mindset		20
	C 2 Professional self-image		21
	C 3 Skills and knowledge		11
	C 4 Influence on personality		16
D *Setting-specific influencing factors*	D 1 Resident-specific factors		29
	D 2 Care process		21
	D 3 Relationship process		45
		D 3/1 Relatives and carers	15
		D 3/2 Resident	
	D 4 Work culture		30

A total of 3 men and 16 women, three (n = 3) from the Vöcklabruck site, eight (n = 8) from the Gmunden site and nine (n = 9) trainees from the Bad Ischl site took part in the study. The average age of the participants (TN) was 33 years for the men (m) and 26 years for the women (f). The interview lasted between 14.57 and 30.49 minutes

(29.81 minutes on average). The preliminary discussion and a follow-up discussion following the interview were not included in the time values. A tabular representation of the sample by allocating the age, gender (f/m) and training centre (BI, GM, VB) of the interviewees can be seen in the following figure. The interview partners (IP) surveyed are anonymised as interviewees B1 to B19, whose statements are shown in italics.

Figure 2: Illustration of the sample

TN	f/m	School	Age	TN	f/m	School	Age
B1	w	BI	26 years	**B11**	w	GM	39 years
B2	w	BI	25 years	**B12**	w	BI	23 years
B3	w	BI	23 years	**B13**	w	BI	26 years
B4	w	BI	24 years	**B14**			
B5	w	GM	45 years	**B15**	w	VB	22 years
B6	w	GM	23 years	**B16**	m	BI	24 years
B7	m	GM	27 years	**B17**	w	GM	23 years
B8	w	BI	21 years	**B18**	w	VB	26 years
B9	w	BI	23 years	**B19**	w	GM	28 years
B10	w	BI	25 years	**B20**	m	GM	49 years

Source: own presentation (postscript of the interviews)

In the following presentation of results, selected findings on the experience of end-of-life care and the factors influencing it are presented. The bullet points represent the categories formed. The results from the transcripts are analysed in more detail on the basis of the subcategories. The line numbers below correspond to the respective paragraph in the transcript.

As the data analysis led to a very extensive collection of results, only the most central results are presented as examples. The frequency of the statements mentioned is not taken into account due to the qualitative research design.

4.1 Experiences in the role as a trainee

Those aspects that particularly characterise the experience are presented in five subcategories. The focus here is on the understanding of the role, expectations, support from carers, theory-practice transfer and the impact on the profession.

4.1.1 Understanding of role

A large proportion of the students surveyed (n = 15) reported several times about a social conflict in their role as a trainee in the context of the nursing interaction process. In the context of their own understanding, this leads to conflicts of conscience and self-doubt, especially when the measures are not in the resident's best interests, as one student reported: "The *carers ordered me to do it, even if the resident didn't like it. Something like a conflict arose in me:* who do *I* do it *for now?"* (B18, 33). Another IP reports something similar: *I wouldn't have done it, but what are you supposed to do as a student, you're always sitting between two chairs when someone orders you to do something and you don't want to do it* (B6, 29).

The trainees are particularly overwhelmed in their role when, as the following statement illustrates, there is an emotional contradiction. *ne could have done something for the resident*, but unfortunately I didn't, and I'm still sorry about that today. Perhaps *more could have been done for the resident (Bi3e38* " (B13, 38).

Not only the execution of the actions, but also one's own attitude can lead to interpersonal conflict. "As a *student, you just do it, even if you would like to do it differently. I couldn't live my own attitude, that was bad."* (B9, 35). Against the background of their knowledge of how to act, learners often perceive a great discrepancy and uncertainty in their behaviour, as the following statements illustrate: *"After I knew that it could be done differently, I* felt *a bit bad about it.*" (B8, 11). *"Ms X had no connection to the church, I knew that because it was in the biography)...). But I wouldn't have dared to tell the ward manager either."* (B6, 31).

Nevertheless, not everyone involved is guided by routine and guidelines, as the following statements confirm: *"When I realised that she no longer wanted to do it, I stopped doing it. I thought to myself that it was expected of me as a student, but if the resident didn't want it, I* wouldn'*t do it/*[(1)] (B13, 14). *"I would have done anything for it. Just because I was a pupil, I didn't realise that I* couldn'*t* be *active if it was* okay.*"* (B15, 21).

4.1.2 Expectations

With the exception of three trainees, all students (n = 16) reported their own expectations. In particular, discussions, active participation, information, dialogue, guidance, support and time were requested. Individual support was particularly emphasised: *"I would have liked more support for myself (...), but also* to be *taken more seriously and* listened to. I would have liked help to *come* when I ask for it.' (B18, 27).

This does not always just mean support in the sense of imparting knowledge, but rather being there and accepting, which the following student emphasises: *"'I just wished that someone would be there to accompany me.* (B3, 41). Often the carers do not even see this need on the part of the trainees: *"I would have liked the carer not to leave me alone. That's what I told her. But she said she didn't think so, she wasn't even aware that I needed support*" (B7, 19).

In addition to personal support, the respondents would have liked to have timely discussions, both in advance to provide information and afterwards for reflection: *"It would have been nice if the carers had told me in advance what end-of-life care is and what it involves,)...) They could also have given us tips for care in a nursing home and told us that all2 nonnal and experienced* /sf." (B12, 43). The role as a student is emphasised again and again: *"As a student in particular, you are confronted with new situations, so the conversation is all the more important."* (B3, 41).

Insufficient sympathy is mentioned as a burden: *"I would have liked a conversation, especially with the first person to die. I was really thrown into water, nobody really took care of me.*" (B18, 45).

Overall, the expectation of active involvement in the counselling is mentioned again and again: *"For me, it was a great wish that I could get actively involved, and I would never have refrained from doing so."* (B15, 19). However, this need is not always honoured: *"I* kept asking to be allowed to be there, but I wasn*'t allowed to or it wasn't addressed.* " (B8, 21).

The trainees also claim to have time after they have completed their training. One student commented: *"I would say that time plays a very important role in learning and feeling the guidance"* (B10, 28). If there is not enough time available for guidance and support, situations are experienced as stressful: *"She just didn't go into the room with me, even though I asked her to. She doesn't have time for that now, she said curtly."* (B6, 9).

4.1.3 Support from carers

In a dual training programme, trainees are accompanied by practice instructors in the practice learning location. Nevertheless, there are differences in support in practice, although this is considered very important by all interviewees (n = 19). Around half of the students surveyed (n = 10) also experienced appropriate support, as one student reported: *"The carers made it possible for me to say goodbye. They also asked me how I was doing. I felt very protected, that helped me a lot."* (B5, 11). During the counselling, empathetic conversations, time and presence were felt to be particularly relieving: *"We talked about it for another half an hour and then I felt better. The conversation was very relieving for me, the nurse even gave me a hug, that was good"* (B11, 11). If carers take care of the trainees and don't leave the students alone, they feel safe in their actions and decisions: "S/he *always explained everything calmly and let me ask lots of questions. She was a real contact person who supported me and took time for me.*" (B19, 31).

Explanations and information about the resident's condition and the dying process are also considered important by the trainees: "I was *very involved in the process of support. I was informed about everything, why and what was being done, why fluids were administered subcutaneously* J." (B2, 31).

Almost 50% (n = 9) felt that keeping the trainees away and marginalising them was stressful. *"The carers didn't even notice, some didn't even realise that we students also have demands and* want to *be actively involved in caring for the dying.*" (B20, 27). It is also often reported that the pupils are not wanted in the support group and *do not need to be there at all. It was alteo SB (Bsch as* mnög//c/7 e/7ed/gt *aB20 unfortunately without* m/ch." (B20, 23). In addition to the lack of involvement of the students in everyday care work, the lack of discussion and sympathy was also experienced as stressful: *"The topic of dying was a taboo subject there, especially when dealing with us students. It was said again and again (...) that someone could die in a care home, but nobody really cared.* " (B6, 7).

The trainees often find it difficult to understand the lack of sympathy and emotionlessness: *"Nobody went into the room with me, not even briefly, nobody took care of me, everyone was so apathetic. That was very incomprehensible to me."* (B18, 23). *"In that case, I was so blanked out as a* student J." (B17, 27).

4.1.4 Theory-practice transfer

At the time of the interviews, all IPs had professional input on end-of-life care in the subject of palliative care. However, only a few students (n = 6) reported a discrepancy between the knowledge they had learnt and their practical actions: "It*'s azmea achwer, if you have dau wiusen dauu, but as a student you can't act the way you should."* (B6, 52). "It *didn't happen the way I learnt about in class, so I was in quite a conflict situation."* (B8, 9). In this context, the trainees also understand the importance of practical implementation, as the following statement confirms: *"The theoretical lessons (...) are an important basis, the practical part has the task of acting as a role model and imparting experiential knowledge.*" (B17, 49).

It is also important for the students to put what they have learnt into practice: *"I really liked* being able to *make suggestions as a trainee, because I already* know what *I want to* do." (B11, 37).

4.1.5 Effects on everyday working life

Some of the students surveyed (n = 12) cited involvement in the support and positive experiences in their interactions as beneficial factors for their later professional life. The active carers have a decisive role model effect, as the following statement confirms: *"The carers have a very important, valuable role model effect in the care of the dying and communication culture. I experienced the optimum in end-of-life care, that was* ec/rf *beautiful."* (B5, 42). The IP continues: *"If I hadn't had such positive experiences in care, then that could trigger a shock experience. Maybe then you avoid such situations (...) where people die."* (B5, 36). Another student commented: "If *you've never learnt it, it's difficult to put it into practice later in your professional life."* (B8, 15). The memory of the first companion or the first dead person usually lasts a lifetime, this is emphasised very often: *"I will always remember my first dead person, it leaves its mark on you. It's also so important that you* have positive experiences, especially with regard to subsequent *mentoring in your professional* life." (B19, 29).

If an appreciative and empathic accompaniment is experienced, the learners' fear of further accompaniment is also taken away: *"I'm not afraid of the next time I have to accompany a dying person, I had a positive experience".* (B4, 38). However, an experience can also be used positively as a negative example and seen as a development process: *"It wasn't a nice experience, but I can take it with me that I will do it differently one day, because it* has to be *done differently."* (B9, 35).

4.2 Emotions in the experience

In addition to the aspects mentioned that apply to the role of the student, emotions are a key aspect of the experience. Different feelings such as sadness, helplessness or fear are reported. Triggering factors and dealing with emotions are also discussed.

4.2.1 Type of emotions

Depending on the patient and the situation, counselling can be perceived as a challenge or a burden. More than half of the students surveyed (n = 12) reported positive and relieving feelings. They reported relief for the person affected: *"I felt relief and was glad that she was allowed to go after fighting for so long."* (B10, 34). The feeling of satisfaction is felt when presence is made possible and needs can be met. *"But it's so nice when you can accompany someone and be there until the end."* (B1, 17). In addition, the sufficient

time spent with the dying person is also decisive for the personal feeling: "*Spending time with the dying person gives me a clear conscience and a satisfying feeling. I have done something that gives the other person pleasure, that they also want."* (B6, 50).

In addition to the acceptance of dying by the resident him/herself, the advanced age is primarily responsible for the feeling of relieving or liberating emotions: *"At the age of 94, you should be allowed to die in peace. That's why I didn't see it as so bad, but as a relief for them."* (B9, 9). As far as the residents are concerned, as the following statement shows, the care is perceived as positive. *"End-of-life care is always very exhausting, but you get a lot in return when someone thanks you. "* (B7, 33).

The emotion of grief (n = 5) is mentioned as one of the most common stressful feelings experienced during care: *"I sat at her bedside, worked for an hour longer (...). Yes, I was sad then, I have to say, it really made me tear up. "* (B11, 11). Furthermore, helplessness (n = 4) and a feeling of powerlessness are very common, according to one pupil: *"It was often the case that I stood there and thought to myself, what should I do now, what should I answer? I was very insecure and felt pretty helpless."* (B13, 8). *"Just having to watch was really hard. I felt so sorry for myself and felt very helpless."* (B4, 14). Fear and feelings of guilt are mentioned very little, more the feeling of pity and insecurity, especially in unpredictable situations: *"(...) and when you go into the room and you see that your breathing is changing at the moment. You think, oh what's happening now, you have an uneasy feeling, but not really fear."* (B7, 29). Trainees report feeling overwhelmed when they find themselves in dialogue situations where they have to answer existential, future-oriented questions: 'I *felt overwhelmed when he said he didn't want to live any more, I didn't know what to say.* (B12, 13).

4.2.2 Triggers for emotions

In addition to the question about possible emotions and how to deal with them, it is also important to answer the question about the factors that trigger them. For one third of the trainees (n = 6), their own preconceptions play a decisive role for the emotion of fear: "*You are afraid of the way the dying person looks, you think and know* a lot." (B1, 14). For a rather large proportion (n = 7), end-of-life care is a completely new situation: *'But I was already afraid to be there at the moment of dying. It would have been a very uncomfortable situation, I didn't want to* be *there.*" (B4, 17).

In addition to the acute confrontation with the phenomenon of dying, passivity is often (n = 8) mentioned as a triggering factor: *"I felt sorry that people just stood there and watched. I myself felt very helpless because of this apathy, but also overwhelmed, I didn't know what I should do."* (B18, 17). In addition to their own wait-and-see attitude, it is also the loneliness of the residents that is perceived as a burden. *"That really hurt me, I don't want to lie alone in a room and die lonely."* (B8, 19). Not only the isolation of the residents, but also being left alone as a student leads to uncertainty and excessive demands, as many students encounter dying people for the first time during their training: *"I was scared when I was alone, otherwise never really."* (B19, 19). In addition, unsatisfactory care by the carers present is experienced as stressful: "After I knew *that it could be different (B8nte, (iB8e iBh me SB8on SB8r felt bad."* (B8, 11).

In the context of care, for some respondentsn = 3), dealing with food and fluids at the end of life is very distressing. On the one hand, this can be the voluntary renunciation of the intake of food and drink, but also the compulsion to eat: *"I also saw that people had to eat, that was very stressful for me."* (B15, 25). The interviewee continued: *"But I also felt helpless when I had to watch someone stop eating. The acceptance of enduring (...) was very difficult for me."* (B15, 39). In addition to the change in food intake, it is also the pain that the trainees find difficult to deal with: "*I felt sorry for the woman, (...) she complained so much about the pain. She cried and screamed every time I touched her. I just didn't understand why she had to* suffer *pain."* (B4, 12).

Shared endurance and the fulfilment of needs are responsible for positive emotions: *"Then I just started crying because I felt so strongly how nice it is (...) that you can accompany someone, that someone is there, that you can still give something."* (B1, 15). If emotions are experienced as pleasing, the trainees even say that they want to be there when she dies: *"(...) because I felt that my presence was good for her. I would have been sad if I hadn't been there when she was dying."* (B11, 33). This statement emphasises the importance of being present and saying goodbye in the process of dying.

4.2.3 Dealing with emotions

Some of the trainees (n = 8) reflect on how to deal with the emotions they have experienced. This revealed a demand for openness. *"The emotions must have a place and have their right to be lived."* (B16, 46). *"You ALSO have to be allowed to say no to people you've grieved for a long time."* (B4, 29). In addition to the emotional confession, confrontation with the situation is also desired if the learners are also aware of its uniqueness: *"Entering the room when you know that a dying person is lying there is always associated with a bit of excitement. But (if you're a23 dri7n2n, old things are half as bad."* (B7, 23). *"But when I was alone, I went into the room despite my insecurity."* (B13, 14).

In addition, it is important to the learners (n = 7) that feelings are allowed and emotions are addressed in everyday care. The emotional expression of crying in particular is relieving and comforting.

One student commented: *"When I was alone and thought about everything, I felt the emotional chaos and everything became too much for me and the tears flowed."* (B16, 39). An individual confrontation is essential for this, as the following statement confirms: *"I think that many people don't know what it's like and that's why they're afraid. Once you face up to this fear, you start to do things differently."* (B1, 34).

However, some of the interviewees not only expressed the desire for closeness and contact, but also the need for distance: *"You need the necessary distance, also a boundary, so that you don't* m/t/e/det *too much."* (B19, 41). In the confrontation and emotional processing, the conversation then offers relief: "*Talking about it is particularly important, (...) that was good. Otherwise I would have felt really bad* if I hadn't been able to share my emotions and thoughts with anyone *(BI2'* (B12, 41).

4.3 Personal factors influencing the experience

In addition to the question about the understanding of the role and the emotions, the personal influencing factors mentioned were one's own attitude, previous experiences, understanding of the profession and personal knowledge.

4.3.1 Attitude and mindset

For the majority of respondents (n = 12), their own attitude as part of their basic personal attitude towards dying and death is an influential factor in their care. The admission of accepting death as a natural process at the end of life is often mentioned: "*But this requires openness, nothing should be tabooed or just accepted. Death is part of life and you can't avoid it.*" (B3, 37). A prerequisite for this is coming to terms with dying and death: "*Consciously coming to terms with it is the prerequisite for humane accompaniment in dying (...), something valuable and supportive for further accompaniment. Otherwise one is afraid and represses things.*' (B9, 43).

If death is accepted, the students feel safe in their actions: "*No, I was never overwhelmed because I accepted the situation as it was. Because death is part of life.*" (B10,20/46). The necessity of confronting the situation of dying people also becomes clear in the following statement: "*(...) anyone who works with life can and should also be able to cope with dying. Dying is a natural thing for me, it will probably happen to all of us.*" (B15, 27/41). Dignity, respect and appreciation are also addressed as an expression of one's own attitude: '*It takes a lot of empathy and feeling from the nursing staff and also an understanding of what is important at the end of life and what is no longer necessary.* (B16, 46).

4.3.2 Experience

Many of the interviewees (n = 13) considered their own previous experience to be a relief: "*(...) I was already there with my grandmother. That was perhaps also the reason that it wasn't so bad for me.*" (B5, 23). *One's own experiences play a major role, namely those already made, including how one grew up with the topic, how one was socialised.*" (B16, 23). Nevertheless, these do not always have an influence on the respective situation: "*Experiences do have an impact, but no death can be compared with another.*" (B19, 35). However, the trainees do not take this experience for granted: "*I'm glad that I was able to experience this for the first time during my training. If you didn't see it all at home (...), I would never have seen it like that.*[1] '(B1, 26).

Frequent confrontations can reduce fear, uncertainty and emotional stress: *"The more dying people I looked after, the more secure I felt."* (B19, 7). *"After I experienced it for the first time, it took away my fear. I didn't know beforehand that it could go so well, although I never had a negative attitude towards it."* (B2, 37). The learners also value the mentoring sequences they experienced, emphasising that experiences are very formative and incisive: *"You become richer in experiences with each mentoring, you learn and grow with the experiences."* (B20, 39). The importance of positive mentoring experiences is always reported: *"The more positive experiences you have, the easier it is"* (B10, 28).

4.3.3 Professional matter of course

Accompanying the dying is part of the core nursing competence, but is not seen as a prerequisite for the profession. However, almost all of the students surveyed (n = 17) are of the opinion that adequate care can definitely be learnt. Empathy and empathy are mentioned as a prerequisite for realising this: *"It's not a prerequisite for the profession, you can learn it. But crying and being sad is part of it. We're not machines, we can't suppress our feelings, nobody can."* (B12, 37). The ability to accompany people in the last hours of life with love and dignity is also seen as a process: *"But you do need a bit of a vocation to be able to accompany people as they die (...). I don't think you can do it in advance, it's something that develops (...). You grow with every accompaniment."* (B11, 19). *A* prerequisite is seen as "*a personal attitude,* vision and *critical* thinking". (B5, 40).

4.3.4 Skills and knowledge

In the context of skills in dealing with the dying, more than 50% of the interviewees (n = 10) reported the importance of theoretically acquired knowledge: *Jn care, nothing was stressful for me, but if I hadn't had the specialised knowledge, it would have been stressful."* (B1, 44). Trainees are required to have knowledge and qualifications, particularly in the area of symptom control: *"I didn't know what to do when she didn't want to eat or drink any more."* (B13,

16). Nevertheless, the students also rely on their feelings and not just on acquired knowledge: "*Caring for the dying has to do with feelings and one's own attitude, not just with specialised knowledge.*" (B7, 39).

4.3.5 Influence on personality

In their experience of end-of-life care, the majority of trainees (n = 10) reported that they became aware of their own transience on the one hand and the special nature of life itself on the other: *"I became more and more aware of my own finiteness and that it can happen very quickly.* " (B4, 15). The care sequences also lead to a more intensive preoccupation and the resulting confrontation with dying and death: "*People also deal with the topic of death in the family, everything is* more open. *The TB1ma is less1)abuised.*" (B19, 41).

The pupils thus appreciate everyday circumstances more again and describe a different approach to life: *"Nothing is taken for granted anymore, you enjoy life more and pay attention to the little things. You* realise *how beautiful UB1* wedvo// *dai (.eben (st.)"* (B12, 49). *"Situations like that bring you back to* the *ground3.*" (B3, 39). In addition to the sustainability of the experiences, it is also about the situation itself: *"It makes something (...). Somehow it slows you down, it's a moment of calm that you feel when you sit there and* shake *hands*." (B17, 41). The trainees also report that they become more self-confident and mature as a result of each individual accompaniment: *"The knowledge and experience I've gained now have helped me grow.*" (B2, 37).

4.4 Setting-specific influencing factors

In addition to the personal aspects, those aspects that are caused by the retirement and nursing home setting also have a significant influence. The main environment-related influencing factors are age, the autonomy of the residents and the relationship and care process.

4.4.1 Work culture

The organisation and observance of a holistic care concept are assigned to the respective work culture of a retirement and nursing home. This is considered particularly important by almost all trainees (n = 14): "If *not dignified end-of-life care in the retirement and nursing home, then where should it happen (...). It's these people's last place, their last home."* (B16, 46).

In addition, the involvement of the residents and the performance of rituals are seen as essential: *"I found the rituals very positive, especially when people died. All the staff wrote cards saying what they wished the deceased (...), that was very nice for me."* (B4, 37).

In the context of the work culture, the requirement to say goodbye is repeatedly mentioned: *"I really wanted to look at her again and wanted to understand death through this. I also really wanted to wash the patient, but unfortunately they said no, the undertaker would do that."* (B8, 11). It is also difficult for the trainees to understand why there is no needs-orientated care or a lack of care: *"They just didn't make any more effort for him, just put liquids on him and did nothing else for him. "* (B9, 33).

The students' experience is also closely linked to the carers' composure: "*I also felt very comfortable because the residents were really treated as people."* (B4, 38). Routine treatments are experienced as very stressful in this respect: *"I think many people just do their programme, they are part of the routine. That's how it should be, that's how we've always done it, they often don't even think about the fact that it's not appropriate in the situation.'* (B17, 25).

4.4.2 Resident-specific factors

Other factors that influence the experience of end-of-life care are those aspects that emanate from the residents themselves. Involvement in decision-making was mentioned several times (n = 8) as an expression of self-determination and independence: *"You want the resident to be well until the end and to be able to make their own decisions. I don't want my decisions to be taken away from me either."* (B2, 17). As long as the residents' self-determination is respected, the trainees find the support very fulfilling: *"I simply asked the person what they wanted and didn't talk them into anything. That's a good and satisfying feeling for you when you know it's in the resident's interest and not something I wanted."* (B11, 29).

Almost all nursing students (n = 18) attach equally high importance to the acceptance of needs through individualised support: *"End-of-life care can be something very nice, doesn't have to be stressful at all, especially not if you can respond to the person."* (B11, 39). *"I responded to them, that was very satisfying for me. I was still able to do what she liked and give her what she preferred, such as beer during oral care. "* (B15, 17).

In addition to the aspects mentioned above, the advanced age of some of the interviewees (n = 6) was also interpreted as a relieving factor: "She has reached *an* age where I thought she could go. That was easier for me (...). But it depends on how the person is doing, whether they *have to suffer or are doing badly, that hurts me too."* (B6, 16). The loneliness of the residents, on the other hand, is experienced as a burden: *"When people are accompanied like this when they are dying, it doesn't feel good. I wish he hadn't always been so alone. I kept going in to see him."* (B9, 35).

4.4.3 Relationship process

Relationship work is discussed in every interview without exception (n = 19) and is therefore very important to all of them. On the one hand, the resident him/herself and, on the other hand, his/her relatives are at the centre of the statements. Accordingly, both perspectives were analysed in a differentiated manner. The relationship with the resident is characterised by closeness, intimacy and familiarity. On the other hand, there is compassion and the difficulty of letting go. *"It really hurt me when she got worse from day to day because I had already taken the resident so close to my heart. When she died, it was really bad. "* (B4, 8).

Against the background of intensive contact, all interviewees (n = 19) reported that for them care is an interactive relationship process: *"The relationship has an emotional influence on the care. If I only know someone briefly, I have access to them (...), to someone I have washed every day, to whom I have told stories and whose life story I* know." (B18, 39). The students attribute the intensity of the contact to the time spent together. Of course, this fact also makes it more difficult to say goodbye and maintain professional distance: *"You know the people more, you learn a lot about them over time. But that doesn't necessarily make it easier, on the contrary, it makes it more difficult."* (B13, 36). The learners also differentiate between dealing with the dying in an acute hospital setting: *"It's different when you've known this person for so long. It's not like in hospital, where you only know them for a short time. I have automatically built up a warm relationship.* When she *died, I suffered with her."* (B4, 10). The pupil continues: *"I couldn't work in a retirement and nursing home (...), I feel so sorry for these people. I would* get *there^a2* zt/g/wde." (B4, 29).

In addition to the intense bond with the dying person themselves, in the context of the relationship work, the contact with relatives and loved ones is mentioned as both a stressful and a relieving factor: *"It was all very bad, I took it very personally, especially the contact with the relatives was bad." (B19, 7).* (B19, 7). The conversation with family members is experienced as a burden if no suitable answers can be found to the questions asked: *"When the relatives were there, I was already overwhelmed. They asked me how she was doing and I didn't know if* I was allowed to *say anything in response*." (B13, 22). *"The worst thing was talking to the relatives. Because when they are so sad, I don't know what to do.*" (B10, 36).

In addition to the feeling of sadness, the majority of students (n = 12) emphasised compassion and empathy: *"I often felt sadness when dealing with relatives, that often hurt the most. Just the way you see everyone standing there and* grieving." (B17, 35). However, when it comes to coping together, the conversation in particular is perceived as relieving and very valuable: *"We talked about how it used to be and how it came about."* (B1, 40). In addition, the shared emotional expression and the presence of the family was perceived as a relief*: "I cried together with my relatives, that was a good and warm feeling."* (B1, 40). *"You know that someone is there and that you're not alone* /often was/ro/7 when anxiety/iönge *dB WBren."* (B7, 37).

4.4.4 Care process

In the care and support of the dying, focussing on the person and their individual needs has top priority and is also mentioned as such by many students (n = 12). A lack of focus on the wishes of the person concerned often leads to stress. The trainees react with a lack of understanding and excessive demands: *"I didn't understand that, he was dying, (...). We let him die of thirst, but we don't have to do anything anymore. We should* force someone to *do something, FOR EXAMPLE.*" (B17, 23). *"It was difficult for me to take measures that simply had to be done, like the body* p/e." (B18, 33). In addition to the nursing challenge, such as administering food and drink, psychosocial circumstances and the question of dying were also perceived as frightening: *"The full body wash was different than usual, normally you attack a warm body where there is still life inside and now the person*'s life *is slowly* fading *away." (B3, 15).* (B3, 15). *"(...) you don't dare to do all that. I was afraid that the resident would die during the camp*." (B12, 25).

In order to negate a confrontation, the students reacted, consciously or unconsciously, by restricting contact: *"After I was so unsure about what I didn't know the answer to the question of wanting to die, I went into the room less. You kind of avoid contact because I didn't know what to say or do."* (B12, 9). If needs-orientated care is practised in the nursing home as part of a palliative farewell culture, the trainees perceive a congruence with their personal values and describe a feeling of satisfaction: *"We wiped her mouth with champagne, (...). She noticed everything, then she took my hand and said thank you very much. I still remember it with great joy today when I can do something GBtes for someone on their last journey. "* (B6, 54).

In order to answer the research questions, the findings of the current research and specialist literature are compared and interpreted in the chapter Discussion.

CHAPTER 5

Discussion and limitation

In the following discussion, the extent to which the results agree with or differ from the specialist literature is analysed. In addition to the interpretations of the statements, an attempt is made to find corresponding explanatory approaches and to uncover accompanying circumstances that may have influenced the results.

5.1 Experiences in the role of trainee

In their role as students, trainees often experience accompanying dying people for the first time (Borasio, 2012; Widegger et al., 2011; Parry, 2011). The results on the experience are in line with the findings of Ohlrogge (2012), who also cites the behaviour of the nursing staff and the role conflict as a student as stressful elements. In line with the studies by Halfpap (2009), Pinho & Barbosa (2010) and Beatty (2013), more than half of the interviewees (n = 15) reported that they had hardly experienced any support and guidance in their day-to-day work. For them, conditions such as having time, having conversations, being allowed to show feelings and receiving information about the resident would be important.

With regard to the lack of support and unsatisfactory communication, one interviewee explained: "*They also (...) didn't ask how you felt about it or how you were doing. Nobody was interested in that.*' (B6, 7). This is often accompanied by an intrarole conflict, as they hardly dare to act independently as students, but want to fulfil the carers' expectations. This results in an emotional dissonance, which Handler (2014) also describes in trained carers and is confirmed by the following statement: "I *always wanted to do everything properly, but the difficult thing was whether I should do it right for the carers or side with the resident.* " (B13, 16).

Similar to Heimerl & Pleschberger (2005), the learners rate the importance of dealing with dying and death and contact with dying people as very high. Unfortunately, however, they are repeatedly discouraged from doing so, especially when the carers themselves are overwhelmed, as one student reported: *"Perhaps the carer was also overwhelmed because she didn't support me at all (ia2)"* (B20, 3). Accordingly, as Wittowski (2012) and Maywald (2014) also state, the teaching of emotional and professional competence in the subject of palliative care is very important, as a third-year trainee emphasises: *"It is also important that it is discussed in class, but that is no substitute for practice. You simply have to* experience *it first-hand as a carer."* (B19, 41). Before the encounter, it is essential to prepare through open and honest communication (Griegoleit, 2011; Rest, 2006).

If there is appropriate guidance and support in everyday life, the trainees can fulfil the tasks assigned to them well. Nevertheless, this study, identical to the findings of Schmidt (2010), confirmed the importance of the role model effect of nursing staff and sensitivity in providing support.

Dealing with the dying can present all those involved with an exceptional professional and personal situation. Terry & Caroll (2008) refer to this as an emotional challenge, which was also confirmed in this study. As Feichtner (2014) also points out, triggering factors can be the first contact and the acute confrontation that takes place. This is aggravated by uncertainty and being left alone, as the following student reports: "It*'s strange when a person lies in front of you who is about to die and you see the whole thing for the first time. But it was clear that she was going to die, but I was already overwhelmed.* " (B3, 11).

The current loneliness of residents, pain situations that cannot be influenced, very complex care situations and dealing with food and fluids in end-of-life care are cited as further reasons for stress and excessive demands (Bausewein, 2004). As also stated in the literature, emotions such as fear, self-doubt, helplessness, anger, sadness, shock and powerlessness are felt (Widegger et al., 2013; Beatty, 2013; Ohlrogge, 2012; Stähli, 2004). However, if person-centred and needs-oriented care is possible, the trainees do not perceive the care as an emotional burden, as one student describes: *"I found out what the dying person valued. Once I knew that, I also knew that I could still do good things and* see a doctor." (B17, 31). The reason for positive, relieving emotions was also demonstrated by Handler (2014), with the author citing feelings such as joy, well-being and satisfaction.

Coping with emotions requires an open and conscious approach to dealing with feelings. Grief, despair, helplessness and powerlessness can be shown, and closeness and distance are allowed. Openness, truthfulness and congruence are named as prerequisites (Engelke, 2015; Beatty, 2013; Lexa, 2011; Griegoleit, 2011; Rest, 2006; Wilkening & Kunz, 2003). The statements in the literature are identical to those of the students. Open and respectful communication as well as showing feelings can be relieving for the situation, especially at the beginning of training, as the following statement shows: "In order to *be able to learn end-of-life care, you have to be allowed and able to allow feelings. To be able to show that you can cry!*" (B12, 39).

5.2 Influencing factors in the experience

Working as an accompanying carer in the dying process offers a constant confrontation with the approaching death. Empathy, empathy and compassion are seen as a professional self-image, but cannot be regarded as a prerequisite (Bischoff-Wanner, 2002). In agreement with Bischoff-Wanner, the interviewees emphasise that end-of-life care can be learned through experience , but can only be carried out with a caring basic understanding and a benevolent sensitivity. *"You can learn how to deal with the dying and how to respond to them if you have cared for a few. You have to have empathy, but you can learn how to deal with them."* (B17, 37). This emphasises the demand for an emotional confrontation through active participation, assistance and the involvement of prospective carers.

All trainees consider their own experience to be an essential factor in dealing with the dying, even if this is often lacking due to their age or the increasing institutionalisation of dying (Ohlrogge, 2012; Borasio, 2012; Aulbert, 2007). The nursing students report that the number of experiences reduces anxiety and gives them confidence in dealing with the situation. One student commented: *"I was already overwhelmed because it was my first work placement and I already had experience of this in the other home."*

(B3, 9). Schwarz-Goavers (2005) emphasises, however, that previous experiences are often applied without reflection and therefore unconsciously guide actions.

Pleschberger and Heimerl (2005) call the accompaniment and care of the dying a "core task" of carers and part of the core nursing skills. In addition to empathy and an understanding of closeness and distance as part of the professional attitude, instruction in professional skills is also required (Griegoleit, 2011; Pleschberger & Heimerl, 2005). The learners emphasise this necessity and see the imparting of skills and knowledge as indispensable, as the following statement emphasises: *"If I hadn't had the skills for this, however, the supervision would have been be1ast4nd. "* (B1,44).

The demand for knowledge and understanding argues for the importance of palliative care as a teaching subject and the need for action in the practice learning environment. A study by Kersting (2005) points to the problem of desensitisation in the practical learning environment. Although the trainees know what they should do, they very quickly orientate themselves to the realities of everyday nursing care. According to , more emphasis should be placed in teaching on the discrepancy between the demand for care of the dying and the actual reality. As a result, training needs to raise awareness by reflecting on and analysing experiences in order to deepen positive experiences and work through negatively perceived situations.

All trainees feel that an appropriate attitude when dealing with the dying is particularly important in connection with their own personality. They cite personal development as being very beneficial as a result of developing an awareness of their own life. *"Accompanying* the dying does something to me. I now enjoy every day, you have to *be aB5tsam and da5kb3)."* (B5, 33).

As stated in the literature, one's own ideas can be shaped and changed by confrontations and experiences (Engelke, 2015; Magon 2014a; Augustyn, 2012). Like the Swiss Professional Association (1990) and the EAPC (Krumm et al., 2015), the target group in this study also affirms the attitude as an expression of respect, dignity, esteem and understanding and demands adherence to these values and norms. For them, the following behaviours must be observed: Death should be accepted as a natural process and emotions must be allowed. The dying person should be treated with respect and treated as a fellow human being.

If these manners are not practised, the support is experienced as very stressful and aggravating, as one student reports: *"It's a shame* that feelings are not taken into account. After all, people should still be *able to feel human,* before aaZern Zn? *Dying."* (B19, 25).

As an influencing factor mentioned several times, the relationship process has an impact on the experience. This means that both the relationship with the resident and with the relatives can represent a challenge. Relationship as a specificity in the long-term care sector is cited several times in the literature and is identical to the results of this study (Raible, 2015; Beatty, 2013; Kränzle, 2011; Müller et al. 2010; Rest, 2006). The development of relationships is confirmed by all of the students surveyed; this can be an expression of closeness and affection and is perceived as both stressful and relieving. The pupils predominantly perceive the relationship as beneficial, only a few as aggravating. In their emotional experience, they differentiate very specifically from the acute sector, in that this factor is rated as much lower in the hospital, as one trainee reports: *"You grieve more when you have a relationship with the resident (...). That was already more than in the hospital, it's really not comparable."* (B2, 25). However, Bauer (2001) points out that the local circumstances and framework conditions should not be held responsible for the relationship as a central element in care, but must always be part of end-of-life care.

The relationship with relatives and loved ones is seen much less as a stressful factor. However, dialogue situations and the feelings of the people present are very much experienced as distressing. If the students are allowed to show their compassion and grief, they experience contact with the family as much less stressful, as Lexa (2011) was also able to prove in her remarks on professional closeness.

In old people's homes and nursing homes, the two most common places for saying goodbye and dying, advanced age, family isolation, lack of independence and multimorbidity are cited as specific characteristics. However, the complexity of chronic illnesses requires dignified support and symptom-orientated care (Engelke, 2015; Bora- sio, 2012; DGP, 2012; Seeger, 2011). As in the surveys in the German nursing home "Rosengarten" by Koch-Straube (1997), in the study on end-of-life care in Saxony (BGW, 2000) and in the study by George (2014), the loneliness and lack of self-determination of the residents is also experienced as very stressful in the context of this research.

Age, on the other hand, is seen as beneficial, as one student explains: *"At 94, you should be allowed to die in peace. That's why I didn't see it as so bad, I saw it as a relief for them."* (B9, 9). If the carers are able to respond to the residents, meet their needs and have time for them, there is never any talk of stress during the visits. Respect for the autonomy of the dying person and the inclusion of the dying person in all nursing activities are of great importance to the students in the care process and are also held responsible for their personal feelings.

In the area of nursing tasks, the interviewees listed the handling of food and fluids, the chronic pain situation and communication with the dying person as situations of excessive demands, as was also documented in the studies by Werner (2013) and Wilkening & Kunze (2003). In particular, helplessness, uncertainty and powerlessness when making decisions about how to proceed are described as stressful. If the trainees feel confronted in this way, they avoid contact and dialogue with the person concerned, often even unconsciously. "If *you simply go in less with a difficult patient, there is automatically less confrontation. You don't feel that way at the time."* (B12, 19). Griegoleit (2011) was also able to demonstrate the aforementioned reduction in contact and delaying behaviour among caregivers who had already received training. In all responses, needs-orientated and activating care was mentioned as one of the most valuable aspects of end-of-life care in connection with the core nursing skills.

The execution of the care actions mentioned and the associated reactions of the carers are closely linked to the working culture practised in the setting. Wilkening & Kunz (2003) call for a

palliative culture of saying goodbye in connection with dying and death. This way of working, characterised by open discussion and individuality, is also desired by the trainees, but is not always experienced. As the retirement and nursing home is the last place of life, respect for quality of life and self-determination are essential factors in terms of holistic care (Giese, 2013). The trainees emphasise the importance of dignified and empathetic encounters and the possibility of rituals when saying goodbye. *"I experienced a dignified and respectful way of dealing with the staff, which was very nice. Dignity and resp38) are important concepts here."* (B5, 38). Nevertheless, the trainees observe that many actions are carried out without questioning them. The students assume that this is due to routine, frustration, insecurity and react with disappointment and pity.

5.3 Limitation

This study is limited in its informative value and limited in some aspects. The age range of 21 to 49 years is very broad, as the 2nd and 3rd year of training was defined as the sample. As a result, there are differences in the previous experiences of the students surveyed in terms of their attitude and understanding of the profession.

Due to the qualitative research approach, the extent and degree of the stress factors were not presented in this study. Further quantitative analysis in the sense of triangulation is required in order to be able to emphasise and illustrate the connection between the individual factors.

The criterion of generalisability in qualitative research processes is not met due to the small population and a sample of 19 students, as the study was only conducted in three nursing schools of one training institution. It would also make sense to have the survey carried out by external researchers in order to rule out any influence from the teacher-student relationship.

Furthermore, the result does not allow for any generalisation to the experience of ster ing in retirement and nursing homes, as the internships took place in different homes and factors such as the age of the trainees or previous experience were not taken into account.

A further limitation of the study can be seen in the analysis of the data, as qualitative research always involves interpretation. The individual categories were assigned inductively and only by the researcher. The comparison of the results, in accordance with the quality criterion of intercoder reliability, by other persons was not possible within the scope of this work (Mayring, 2010, p. 117). Therefore, the allocation to the categories is very subjective, which means that the scientific quality criteria of objectivity and reliability could not be fully met (Mayer, 2007, p. 99).

The criterion of intracoderiability was met by prior manual coding and a subsequent, computer-assisted, threefold and time-shifted material run-through (Ma- yring, 2010, p. 117).

A communicative validation of the results was only carried out with three pupils at the Bad Ischl school site.

CHAPTER 6

Summary and conclusion

To date, only a few results are available in German-speaking countries on the experience of providing end-of-life care in nursing training. In particular, there is a lack of concrete results on dealing with the dying in the setting of retirement and nursing homes. The aim of this research work was to present a comprehensive picture of the care of the dying from the perspective of the trainees and to filter out those factors that have a relieving or stressful influence on the care.

The results in the statements on the experience as a trainee show that the trainees experience their role as a student very differently. Supporting the dying is often driven by a conflict of intraroles and emotional dissonance and is strongly influenced by their own expectations.

Assistance is experienced as very person- and situation-dependent. This becomes a burden if there is a lack of support from carers, if the person's own emotions are not allowed to be shown and if the dying person's needs are not respected as an individual and a human being. The trainees would like to receive appropriate support and guidance, especially during their first contact with the dying.

The trainees also do not always feel recognised as carers and therefore often act very cautiously and with little self-determination in their actions. The working culture of the institution and the relationship with the resident are key influencing factors in the context of emotional experience. Emotional feelings centre primarily on grief, powerlessness, helplessness and pity. The term "excessive demands" is used when there is no adequate support and a lack of confrontation with dying and death.

Personal attitudes and one's own previous experiences play a decisive role in the question of influencing factors. Experiences must be worked through by reflecting on and analysing the situations experienced. Accompanying the dying is not a professional matter of course, but it can be learnt with the appropriate social and emotional skills and have a lasting influence on awareness. Particularly in the setting of retirement and nursing homes, the advanced age of the residents is a relieving factor, but the relationship process is a stressful one.

In order to prepare students for the confrontation with dying and death in the long-term care sector, sufficient support and guidance is required during training. Dealing with one's own experiences and processing the emotions experienced must be considered part of the training. The existence of experience with end-of-life care should not be taken for granted.

Accordingly, sufficient support is required from carers in practice and teachers in the classroom. Existing fears, emotional stress factors, helplessness and feelings of powerlessness must be taken into account in training in order to support a palliative attitude and achieve emotional competence. Apart from the intrinsic burden, end-of-life care can lead to personal satisfaction, professional success and individual personal development if these criteria are taken into account.

The researcher and author of this work was able to verify her observation and hypothesis that accompanying the dying is only a burden if there is no corresponding support from carers. New insights were gained into the validity of relationship work and the importance of self-determination. The importance of emotional work was thus further emphasised by examining and analysing the support experienced.

The results of this study could be used for further education and training programmes or for presentation at specialist conferences. Nursing staff in practice would then find it easier to understand the situation of the trainees or to empathise with their role . Nursing educators, practice instructors and nursing service managers could find impulses for optimal support and then implement these in their guidance of trainees.

CHAPTER 7

Conclusion and outlook

The analysis of the data collected and the subsequent processing of the results have shown that the new findings largely correspond to the aspects presented in the literature review.

Only the stress factors could be identified in this study. The extent to which these factors play a role in overload in everyday working life could be the subject of a further study. A comparative study would also be interesting in order to answer the question of whether trainees experience end-of-life care differently in retirement and nursing homes than in hospitals. In terms of skills development, the experience at the beginning and the experience at the end of training could also be compared and the effect of death education analysed. The amendment of the nursing training programme and its transfer to the tertiary education sector poses new challenges for all those involved. Due to the increased number of students in the classroom, the changed allocation of teaching hours for the subject of palliative care and the demand for self-learning skills, up-to-date didactic methods are required to convey attitudes, values and standards in a sustainable manner. In the interests of all those affected, this requirement must be met through openness in dealing with the phenomenon of dying, through an emotional approach and through appropriate support in practice. This requires a holistically orientated understanding of care in schools and a palliative culture of dying in practice. The promotion of a farewell culture attitude among nursing students requires sensitisation in the context of dealing with the reality of death and one's own finiteness, as well as reflection on existing factors of interaction with the dying.

CHAPTER 8

Bibliography

Albrecht, E. (2010). The dying process. In Bausewein, C., Roller, S. & Voltz, R (eds.). Guide to palliative care. Palliative medicine and hospice care (pp. 522-526). Munich: Urban & Fischer Verlag.

Araujo M., Silva M., Francisco M. (2004). Nursing the dying: essential elements in the care of terminally ill patients. International Nursing Rev, 51/3, 149-158.

Aulbert, E. (2007). Communication with patients and relatives. In Aulbert, E.; Nauck, F. & Radbruch, L. (Eds.). Textbook of palliative medicine (p. 10681089). Stuttgart & New York: Schattauer Verlag.

Andraschko, H. G. (2008). Palliative care. Project and quality management in healthcare.available at http://www.pqm- online.de/download/palliativpflege [27.07.2016].

Bauer, R. (2001). Basis of nursing relationship work. Psychologie Pflege, vol. 7, 309-314.

Bausewein, C., Roller, S. & Voltz, R. (2010). Guide to palliative care. Palliative medicine and hospice care. Munich: Urban & Fischer Verlag.

Beatty, I. (2013). End-of-life care from the perspective of students in basic nursing training. Bern: Hep-Verlag.

Beutel, H. (2011). Psychosocial support for the dying and their relatives. In Kränzle, S./ Schmid, U./Seeger, C. (eds.), Palliative Care. Handbook for care and support (pp. 33-38). Berlin/Heidelberg: Springer Verlag.

BGW (German Social Accident Insurance Institution for the Health and Welfare Services) (2010). Research results of the study "End-of-life care in Saxony". Work and stress situation of carers and doctors. Hamburg.

Bioethics Commission (2015). Dying with dignity. Recommendations on the accompaniment and care of people at the end of life and related issues. Statement by the Bioethics Commission, Federal Chancellery, Vienna.

Borasio, G.D. (2012). About dying. What we know, what we can do, how we prepare for it. Munich: Beck Verlag.

Boeree, G. (2006). Personality theory - Abraham Maslow. Shippensburg University, USA. Available at http://www.social-psychology.com/do/PT_maslow.pdf [25 July 2016].

Brisley P, Wood L. (2004). The impact of education and experience on death anxiety in new graduate nurses. *Contemp Nurse,* 17, 102-108.

Bischoff-Wanner, C. (2002). *Empathy in nursing.* Bern: Hans Huber Verlag.

Charalambous, A., Kaite, C. (2013). Undergraduate nursing students cringing for cancer patients: hermeneutic phenomenological insights of their experiences. BMC Health Services Research, 13:63. 1-13. available at http://bmchealthservres.biomedcentral.com/articles/10.1186/1472-6963-13-63 [20.08.2016].

Cooper, J. & Barnett, M. (2005). Aspects of caring for dying patients which cause anxiety to first year students. *International Journal of Palliative Nursing, 11*, 423-430.

Dasch, B., Blum, K., Gude, P. & Bausewein, C. (2015). Place of death: trends over the course of a decade - a population-based study of death certificates from the years 2001 and 2011. Deutsches Ärzteblatt, 112, 496-504. DOI: 10.3238/arztebl.2015.0496.

Davies, E. & Higginson I.J. (2008). The solid facts - Palliative care. WHO Europe. Available at http://www.euro.who.int/__data/assets/pdf_file/0009/98235/E82933.pdf [02.08.2016].

DGP (German Society for Palliative Medicine) (2010). Charter for the care of seriously ill and dying people in Germany.

DGP (German Society for Palliative Medicine) (2012). Policy paper on the development of "Hospice culture and palliative care in inpatient facilities for the elderly. Care of seriously ill and dying people of advanced age in care facilities.

DGP (German Society for Nursing Science e.V. (n.d.). Belmont Report. Available at: http://www.dg-pflegewissenschaft.de/pdf/Belmont- Report.pdf [20/08/2016].

Ek, K. et al (2014). Death and caring for dying patients: exploring first-year students' descriptive experiences. *International Journal of Palliative Nursing,* 20, 509-515, doi: 10.12968/ijpn.2014.20.10.509.

Engelke, E. (2015). *The truth about dying*. Munich: Rowohlt Verlag GmbH.

Engelke, E. (2013). Those who want to accompany the dying must allow themselves to be guided by them. *Nursing journal, vol. 66*, 6-7.

Feichtner, A. (2014). *Textbook for palliative care.* Vienna: Facultas publishing house.

Feichtner, A. (2016). *Palliative care in practice, knowledge and application.* Vienna: Facultas publishing house.

Flick, U. (2012). *Qualitative social research. An introduction.* Reinbeck: Rowohlt publishing house.

Gerhard, C. (2015). Practical knowledge of palliative care. Concepts for a wide range of palliative care situations. Stuttgart: Thieme publishing house.

George, W. (2014). Dying in inpatient care facilities, In George, W. (2015). Heterogeneous quality in inpatient facilities, Pflegezeitschrift, vol. 68, 652-656.

Gero, R.J. & Zimbardo, P.G. (2008). Psychology.

Giese, C. (2013). Being able to die one's own death. Care in the last phase of life, Pflegezeitschrift, vol. 66, 15-18.

Gläser, J. & Laudel, G. (2010). Expert interviews and qualitative content analysis. Wiesbaden: VS Verlag für Sozialwissenschaften.

Griegoleit, U. (2011). Dealing with dying and death in the hospital institution. On the development of a farewell-cultural attitude in nursing training. Frankfurt/Main: Peter Lang Verlag.

Göckenjan, G. (2008). Dying in our society - ideals and realities. In Federal Agency for Civic Education (ed.): Aus Politik und Zeitgeschichte. Death and dying.

GuK-AV (1999): Health and Nursing Training Ordinance. Ordinance of the Federal Minister of Labour, Health and Social Affairs on training in the higher service for health care and nursing. Available at https://www.ris.bka.gv.at/Geltende Fassung.wxe?Abfrage= Bundesnormen&Gesetzesnummer=10011179 [12.07.2016].

Halbmayr-Kubicsek, U. (2015). Meeting death and dying - Fears and expectations of health and nursing students regarding future confrontation with dying and death, Pflegewissenschaft, vol. 11, 596-603.

Handler, S. (2014). Emotion work in end-of-life care. Nursing Science, vol. 16, 210-224.

Halfpap, N. (2009). When *patients die - how nurses deal with death and grief.* University Medical Centre Freiburg i. Breisgau. Available at https://www.freidok.uni-freiburg.de/dnb/download/6896 [09.07.2017].

Hausmann, C. & Koller, M. (2011). *Psychology, sociology and pedagogy. A textbook for nursing and healthcare professions.* Vienna: Facultas publishing house.

Heimerl, K. et al. (2000). Maintaining autonomy: a qualitative patient survey in home nursing. In Seidl, E; Stankova, M. & Walter, I. (eds.): Autonomy in old age. Studien zur Verbesserung der Lebensqualität durch professionelle Pflege, *Pflegewissenschaft heute,* Vol. 6, Vienna: Maudrich Verlag, pp. 102-165.

Heimerl, K. (2007). Needs of patients and residents at the end of life. In Knipping, C. (Ed.), *Textbook Palliative Care* (pp. 131-138). Bern: Verlag Hans Huber.

Heller, A. & Knipping, C. (2007). Palliative care - attitudes and orientations. In Knipping, C. (Ed.), *Lehrbuch Palliative Care* (pp. 39-47), Bern: Verlag Hans Huber.

Heller, A. et al. (2007): Palliative culture in inpatient care for the elderly. In Heller, A; Heimerl, K. & Husebo, S.: Wenn nichts mehr zu machen ist, ist noch viel zu tun. Freiburg: Lambertus Verlag.

Hochschild, A. (2006). *The bought heart. The commercialisation of emotions.* Frankfurt am Main: Campus Bibliothek.

Hospice Austria (2010). Palliative geriatrics. Brief information on the curriculum for employees of retirement and nursing homes.

Available at http://www.hospiz.at/pdf_dl/Kurzinfo_Curriculum_Palliative_Geriatrie.pdf [18/08/2016].

ICN Code of Ethics for Carers (2012). Available at https://www.pflege-charta.de/fileadmin/charta/Arbeitshilfe/Modul_5/M5-ICN-Ethikkodex- DBfK_.pdf [11.07.2017].

Jafari, M. (2015). Caring for dying patients: attitude of nursing students and effects of education. International Journal of Palliative Nursing, 21, 192-197, doi: 10.4103/0973-1075.156497.

Kessler, D. (1997). The rights of the dying, Weinheim: Beltz Verlag.

Kersting, K. (2005). The situation of nursing students: Aspiration and reality, Pflegepädagogik, vol. 07, 31-37.

Koch-Straube, U. (1997). Foreign world nursing home. Reports from an ethnological study. Pflege Gesellschaft, vol. 02, 7-10.

Kostrzewa, S. & Kutzner, M. (2002). What we can still do! Basal stimulation in end-of-life care. Bern/Göttingen/Toronto/Seattle: Verlag Hans Huber.

Kössler, H. (2016). *Consequences of the GuKG - Amendment 2016 BGBl. I No. 75/2016* for the general and specialised palliative and hospice sector. Available at http://www.hospiz-baden.at/wp-content/uploads/2016/09/GuKG-Novelle-2016.pdf [06.07.2017].

Kränzle, S. (2011). When nothing more can be done - The beginning of therapy is the beginning of palliative care. In Kränzle, S./ Schmid, U./Seeger, C. (eds.), *Palliative Care. Handbook for care and support* (pp. 20-21). Berlin, Heidelberg: Springer Verlag.

Krumm, N., Schmidlin, E., Schulz, C. & Elsner, F. (translated , 2015): Core competences in palliative care - a white paper from the European Association for

Palliative Care on teaching palliative care. First publication: Gamondi, C., Larkin, P. & Payne, S.: Core competencies (2013): a palliative care education - part 1, *Journal of Palliative Medicine, 16,* 152165, doi: 10.1055/s-0035-1552684.

Kuckartz, U. (2016). *Qualitative content analysis. Methods, practice, computer support.* Weinheim/Basel: Beltz Juventa Verlag.

Kunz, R. (2007). Holistic assessment as the basis of palliative care in geriatrics. In Knipping, C. (Ed.), *Textbook Palliative Care* (pp. 124130). Bern: Verlag Hans Huber.

Kühne-Ponesch, S. (2004). *Models and theories in nursing.* Vienna: Facultas Verlag.

Kübler-Ross, E. (2013). *Interviews with the dying.* Freiburg: Kreuz Verlag.

Lamnek, S. (2010). *Qualitative social research.* Weinheim/Basel: Beltz Verlag.

Lampert, B. (2011). Good care needs closeness and distance at the same time. Available at http://www.pressetext.com/news/20111216004 [18.08.2016].

Lexa, N. (2011). Professional closeness instead of professional distance. *pflegen: palliativ, vol. 10,* 20-22.

Magon, H. (2014a) Fears and needs of seriously ill and dying people, part 1. *Zeitschrift für Palliativmedizin, vol. 15*, 94-99.

Magon, H. (2014b) Fears and needs of seriously ill and dying people, Part 2. *Journal of Palliative Medicine, Vol. 15*, 154-157.

May, A. (2011). When nothing more can be done - The beginning of therapy is the beginning of palliative care. In Kränzle, S./ Schmid, U./Seeger, C. (eds.), Palliative Care. Handbook for care and support (pp. 21-29). Berlin/Heidelberg: Springer Verlag.

Mayer, H. (2007). Pflegeforschung anwenden, Elemente und Basiswissen für Studium und Weiterbildung. Vienna: Facultas publishing house.

Mayring, P. (2002). Introduction to Qualitative Social Research. A guide to qualitative thinking, Weinheim & Basel: Beltz Verlag.

Mayring, P. (2010). Qualitative Content Analysis. Basics and techniques, Weinheim

& Basel: Beltz Verlag.

Maywald, C. (2014). The pedagogical handling of dying, death and grief. Teaching, counselling and support, Hamburg: Disserta Verlag.

Monteverde, S. (2007). Ethics & Palliative Care - The Good as an Orientation for Action. In Knipping, C. (Ed.), Textbook Palliative Care (pp. 520-535). Bern: Verlag Hans Huber.

Moser, H. (2012). Toolbox for practical research. An introduction. Freiburg im Breisgau: Lambertus Verlag.

Müller-Busch, H.C. (2013). Farewell takes time. Palliative care and the ethics of dying. Berlin: Suhrkamp Verlag.

Müller-Busch, H.C. (2014). Palliative Care - History and concept of interdisciplinary care for the seriously ill and dying. Ethics Journal, vol. 2, 1-16.

Müller, M., Pfister, D., Markett, S. & Jaspers, B. (2010). How much death can the team tolerate. A nationwide survey of palliative care units in Germany. Journal of Palliative Medicine, vol. 11, 227-233. doi: 10.1055/s-0030-1248520.

Nagele, S. & Feichtner, A. (2012). Textbook of palliative care. Vienna: Facultas Verlag.

National Ethics Council. Self-determination and care at the end of life, statement (2006). Berlin. Available at http://www.ethikrat.org/dateien/pdf/selbstbestimmung-und-fuersorge-am- lebensende.pdf [25.07.2016].

Ohlrogge, C. (2012). Dealing with dying people from the perspective of trainees in nursing professions. Unpublished Master's thesis, Faculty of Nursing and Health Sciences, Protestant University of Applied Sciences, Darmstadt.

Parry, M. (2011). Student nurses experience of their first death in clinical practice. International Journal of Palliative Nursing, 17/9, 446-453.

Peplau, H. (1995). Interpersonal relationships in nursing. Kassel: Recom Verlag.

Pinho, L.M.O, Barbosa, M.A. (2010). The professor-student relationship in coping with dying, In. Revista da Escola de Enfermagem da USP, 44, 106111.

Pleschberger, S., Heimerl, K. & Wild, M. (2005). Teaching and learning palliative care. The care of seriously ill and dying people in the context of nursing training programmes. In Pleschberger, S., Heimerl, K. & Wild, M. (Eds.), Palliative care. Fundamentals for practice and teaching (pp. 15-29). Vienna: Facultas Verlag.

Pleschberger, S. (2005). Just don't be a burden. Dying with dignity from the perspective of elderly people in nursing homes. Freiburg im Breisgau: Lambertus Verlag.

Pribil, U. (2005). The last hours - accompanying and caring for dying people. In Pleschberger, S., Heimerl, K. & Wild, M. (Eds.), Palliative care. Basics for practice and teaching (pp. 189-200). Vienna: Facultas Verlag.

Raible, W. (2015). Support until the end. Experiences and help in accompanying dying people. Freiburg im Breisgau: Herder Verlag.

Rest, F. (2006). Assisted dying, end-of-life care, end-of-life counselling. Handbook for inpatient and outpatient care. Stuttgart: Kohlhammer Verlag.

Seeger, C. (2011). Guidelines for palliative care. In Kränzle, S./ Schmid, U./Seeger, C. (Eds.), Palliative Care. Handbook for care and support (pp. 9-14). Berlin, Heidelberg: Springer Verlag.

Schwarz-Goavers, R. (2005). Subjective theories as a basis for knowledge and action. Nursing didactic conclusions for learning field and problem-orientated teaching. PflegePädagogik, vol. 01, 38-49.

Schmidt, D. (2010). Encountering dying and death. How learners can be supported. Die Schwester, Der Pfleger, vol. 49, 642-647.

Stähli, A. (2004). Dealing with emotions in palliative care. A guide. Stuttgart: Kohlhammer Verlag.

Steffen-Bürgi, S. (2011). Reflections on selected definitions of palliative care. In Knipping, C. (Ed.), Textbook Palliative Care (pp. 30-38). Bern: Verlag Hans Huber.

Steinke, I. (2000). Quality criteria of qualitative research. In Flick, U. et al. (eds.): Qualitative Research. A handbook (pp. 319-331). Reinbek near Hamburg: Rowohlt

Verlag.

Stigler, H. & Felbinger, G. (2005). The interview guide in the qualitative interview. In Stigler, H. & Reicher, H. (Eds.). Praxisbuch Empirische Sozialforschung in den Erziehungs- und Bildungswissenschaften (pp. 129-134). Innsbruck: Studienverlag.

Student, J.C., Mühlum, A., Student, U. (2004). Social work in hospice and palliative care. Munich: Reinhardt. UTB Verlag.

Stöhr, M. & Trumpetter, N. (2006). Developing a professional self-image and learning to cope with professional demands. Vienna: Urban & Fischer Verlag.

Terry, L.M. & Carroll, J. (2008). Dealing with death: first encounters for first- year nursing students. British Journal of Nursing, 17, 760-766.

Thielhorn, U. (2005). Nursing theories and quality development in palliative care. In Pleschberger, S., Heimerl, K. & Wild, M. (Eds.), Palliative care. Fundamentals for practice and teaching (pp. 67-77). Vienna: Facultas Verlag.

Vogt, S. (2010). Palliative care in nursing homes - time and attention are elementary. Journal of Palliative Medicine, Vol. 13, DOI: 10.1055/s-0030- 1249717.

Wasner, M. (2013). Do not overlook the needs of the dying and their relatives Nursing journal, vol. 66, 10-13.

Watzlawick, P. et al. (1990). Human communication. Verlag Hans Huber: Bern/Göttingen/Toronto/Seattle.

Werner, S. (2013). "We can't let anyone starve". Food and fluid intake at the end of life. Nursing journal, vol. 66, 30-33.

Weiss-Faßbinder, S. & Lust, A. (2017). Health and Nursing Care Act - *GuKG.* Vienna: Manzsche Verlags- und Universitätsbuchhandlung.

Widegger, S., Schulc, E. & Them C. (2011). Emotional work in end-of-life care, A quantitative exploratory study to survey the emotional work of qualified health and nursing staff in end-of-life care. Nursing Science, vol. 02, 100-112.

Wilkening, K. & Kunz, R. (2003). Dying in the nursing home. Perspectives and practice of a new culture of farewell. Göttingen: Vandenhoeck & Ruprecht Verlag.

CHAPTER 9

Appendix

9.1 Appendix 1 Written questionnaire

Dear student,

As part of the university course in palliative care at the PMU Salzburg, I am writing my final thesis on the topic of "Between the fronts": end-of-life care in long-term inpatient care from the perspective of nursing students.

In order to draw up the interview guidelines as part of qualitative research, I would like to ask about the experience of dying and death from the perspective of nursing students on their practical training in retirement and nursing homes. In doing so, you can make a significant contribution to including those aspects in the interview guide that you have experienced as a trainee.

The questionnaire is of course anonymous and is only accessible to the researcher for the purpose of the study. Please write down your comments on the following sheet.

How did you experience accompanying dying people as a carer in a retirement and/or nursing home?

Describe a situation that you experienced. The sub-questions are only intended to support your thoughts. I ask you to answer openly and honestly.

- What was the encounter with dying people like for you?
    - How was the contact with the elderly person?
    - How did it make you feel?
    - Was there anything that was particularly stressful, that you were afraid of?
- What tasks did you carry out?
    - Was there anything you found particularly difficult?
- What uncertainties arose when accompanying dying people?
    - Communication, feelings, relatives

Thank you very much for your co-operation.

9.2 Appendix 2 Conducting the interview

A guided interview was chosen for the data collection. The students actively have their say and first answer the narrative-generating question. They report on their experiences of dealing with dying and death in retirement and nursing homes. At the beginning, is asked an introductory question about the location of the internship, followed by the narrative-generating question as an open question,

Procedure of the interview

Greeting the student,

Hello, Mrs/Mr Thank you for volunteering to conduct this interview with me. I am conducting the interview as part of a research project in the expert course for palliative care at the PMU Salzburg.

Information on conducting the interview

I will read you the signed consent form again and ask you to confirm with yes or to answer no.

- Are you taking part in the interview voluntarily?
- You have been informed in writing and verbally by me as the researcher about the conditions of participation in the interview?
- You have received sufficient information about the interview procedure.
- Are you aware that the data will be published for research purposes but will be anonymised?

Information on speaking behaviour, recording, time frame, anonymity

- You may take as long as you like to answer the questions
- You should answer the questions asked honestly and authentically and ask questions if anything is unclear.
- You know that you have the right to interrupt at any time and that you cannot be forced to take part in the interview?
- The interview will be recorded using a tape recorder and then transcribed anonymously in writing. The data can only be viewed by the researcher.

9.3 Appendix 3 Interview guide

Introductory question: How old are you? In which care or nursing home were you confronted with dying and death?

Narrative-generating question: How did you experience the encounter with dying people as a carer in a retirement or nursing home?

Topic area 1 - Nursing challenges

Which caring activities were a challenge for you?

Can you name specific situations where you were overwhelmed with caring for the dying?

How did you experience caring for relatives and carers?

Were there situations where you were unsure of what to do? Why was that?

What influence did the relationship with the resident have?

Subject area 2 - Emotional experiences

What positive and negative feelings did you experience when caring for the dying?
What was the trigger for these feelings, why did you feel them?
Was there anything you were afraid of?

Topic 3 - Expectations of the care profession

Were your personal expectations fulfilled in the care of the dying in a retirement and nursing home?
Did you experience caring for the dying as a professional matter of course?
What can you take away for yourself from this support?
What else would you have needed or wished for?
How did you experience your role as a trainee?

Topic area 4 - Analysing the environment of the retirement and nursing home

What did you find **disturbing or helpful on** the part of the retirement **and nursing home** ....?
What did you experience as supportive or stressful on the part of the carers providing instruction?

Kolibri 360 GmbH
Ferdinand-Jühlke-Straße 7
99095 Erfurt, Deutschland
produktsicherheit@kolibri360.de

Druck:
CPI Druckdienstleistungen GmbH
im Auftrag der
Kolibri 360 GmbH
Ferdinand-Jühlke-Str. 7
99095 Erfurt